Praise for *Therapy Revolution*

"Don't let its accessible language fool you—this book is packed with salient information rooted in a solid sense of ethics. As the medical director of a psychiatric hospital, I believe that this book not only has an important place on the shelf of therapy patients but would also be valuable reading for any professional, instructor, or student in the fields of mental health and addiction. *Therapy Revolution* will likely be relevant for years to come."

—Jeffrey Borenstein, M.D., CEO and Medical Director,
Holliswood Hospital, Holliswood, NY

"This book has been an ambitious undertaking. And, well worth the effort! It is methodical, well structured, thorough, and easy to understand. The metaphors and analogies are superb, and help greatly in clarifying the ideas the authors wish to convey.

"As a retired clinical psychologist with many years of clinical experience, I really enjoyed reading this book. I think that it will be useful not only to those who are eager to find a competent psychotherapist and a better understanding of what psychotherapy is all about, but even to practicing psychotherapists."

—John Hoffman, Ph.D., Retired Clinical Psychologist,
Formerly of Veterans Administration Center, Buffalo, NY

"Timely! The public needs a book like this. Richard and C.R. Zwolinski have accomplished their task with clarity, thoroughness, and passion. This book will help you pick a competent therapist and receive the treatment you need and deserve. Not only a must-read for the intelligent consumer, but a practical guide and useful resource for the therapist as well!"

—John Eppolito, Clinical Psychologist
Illinois Youth Center, St. Charles, Illinois

"As a psychiatrist, I know how important it is to work with experienced and ethical psychotherapists. *Therapy Revolution* is an eye-opener—it shows what can go wrong in therapy, and how to avoid it. It really gives the reader tools with which to evaluate a therapist and get the best care possible without wasting time or money. I highly recommend this book to patients, their families, to psychotherapists, and to anyone who must make a referral to a therapist."

—Lyubov Gorelik, M.D., Psychiatrist

THERAPY REVOLUTION

Find Help, Get Better, and Move on
without Wasting Time or Money

Richard M. Zwolinski, LMHC, CASAC
and C. R. Zwolinski

Health Communications, Inc.
Deerfield Beach, Florida

www.hcibooks.com

THIS BOOK IS DEDICATED

TO THERAPY PATIENTS

EVERYWHERE.

Library of Congress Cataloging-in-Publication Data

Zwolinski, Richard M.
    Therapy revolution : find help, get better, and move on without wasting time or money
/ Richard M. Zwolinski and C.R. Zwolinski.
      p. cm.
    Includes bibliographical references and index.
    ISBN-13: 978-0-7573-1418-6
    ISBN-10: 0-7573-1418-X
    1. Psychotherapy—United States. 2. Psychotherapists—United States.
  3. Psychotherapy—Practice—Evaluation. I. Zwolinski, C. R. II. Title.
    RC480.5.Z86 2009
    616.89'14—dc22   2009027419

Publisher: Health Communications, Inc.
        3201 S.W. 15th Street
        Deerfield Beach, FL 33442–8190

Cover design by Larissa Hise Henoch
Interior design and formatting by Lawna Patterson Oldfield

Contents

Acknowledgments

We are blessed with many colleagues and friends who have been a source of inspiration. John Hoffman, Ph.D., teacher, mentor, and psychologist par excellence, who read and commented on the manuscript and suggested the important addition on psychodrama. Barry Strauss, Ph.D., author and historian, who not only read the manuscript but also encouraged us to write a book about therapy in the first place. We benefited greatly from his advice and enthusiasm. John Eppolito, Psy.D., who reviewed the manuscript and gave important feedback.

Without the unfailing support, sage advice, and kindness of our dear friend Bracha Klein (and her family), this book might never have been written. Thank you.

Thanks to all the dedicated experts at New York State OASAS, including Charles Monson, William Lachanski, Joseph Chelales, Patricia Lincourt, Steven Rabinowitz, and their colleagues. They have all had an influence on this book. Dick Gallagher, Executive Director of Alcohol and Drug Dependency Services, and Gerry Erion deserve thanks for raising treatment standards and delivering compassionate and effective care. Kathy Adamson, Jennifer Aromanda, Beverly Berkowitz, Lyubov Gorelik, M.D., Gay Hartigan, Maria Mootoo, Sultan Niazi, John Neikirk, George Ryer, Michele Saari, Stephanie Scotti, Patrice Wallace-Moore, and Roy Wallach of Arms Acres all deserve our thanks.

Many people help shape our thoughts and beliefs about personal and professional ethics as well as enrich our lives with personal and professional relationships, including: Nigel Ashley, Dov Berdy, Rabbi Shalom Blatter, Jacques Doueck, D.D.S. and his team, Yehuda Farkas, the Fleischer Family, Basha Genova Freedman, Kelly Garrity-Jackson, our dear friend Harold Glickstein, John Guyette, G. T. Jakubovics, Spencer Johnson, Jr., the Katz family, Steven and Alicia Ludwig, John Mercurio, Wilbur Mills, Marcia Mogelonsky, L. Salzberg, Tamer Seckin, M.D., Rivkah Slonim, Chuck D. Stevens, Rabbi Binyamin Stimler, Dovid and Dena Taub, Oleg and Vicky Tselnik, Lena Warr, and Timothy Welsh.

The Fischman family has opened their joyful home to us for nearly five years—we are very grateful. The witty Stacie Orell and gentleman and cartoonist Mark Hill are always helpful. James Fox, CEO of Vigilar, inspires us with his creativity and drive. We are indebted to literary agent Cathy Hemming, who generously gave us so much of her time and invaluable advice about the world of books and publishing. Rabbi Abraham Twerski, M.D., gave us permission to use part of his excellent book, *Generation to Generation*. Dr. Wah Lee, D.O., and Ellen Gordon, Feldenkrais practitioner, helped heal computer-related aches and pains.

Thanks to our editor Michele Matrisciani, and the HCI team, including publisher Peter Vegso, Carol Rosenberg, Larissa Hise Henoch, Candace Johnson, Kim Weiss, Lawna Patterson Oldfield, Justin Rotkowitz, Jaron Hunter, Nicole Haye, and Tonya Woodworth. We are grateful for the expertise of our developmental editor Natasha Graf and the enthusiasm of copy editor Cathy Slovensky.

We must thank our literary agent Scott Gould at RLR Associates for *everything*. We feel blessed to have found you.

We are indebted to all the former and current therapy patients who shared their personal stories with us and allowed us to use their stories in this book. Thank you from the bottom of our hearts for your trust.

We are blessed with a warm and understanding family: Mom (Josephine Zwolinski Glaser) and brothers Robert and William. Dad (Stanley Zwolinski, 1917-1972) taught all his children to always do the right thing.

We humbly acknowledge our ever-present gratitude to God, who gives each one of us challenges to grow from and missions to fulfill. We hope that this book fulfills part of ours.

Introduction

There is an unnamed crisis in America today that is affecting as many as one in four Americans. Psychotherapy as we know it is failing to help many who turn to it for help. At best, many people who have been in therapy say it just isn't worth the money. At worst, they say they are confused and have been hurt by the experience. And make no mistake about it, like physical medical malpractice, botched or incompetent psychotherapy can exacerbate a patient's suffering, causing very real and lasting damage. We call this problem the "therapy crisis," and we hope this book will be part of the solution.

A national study conducted by the U.S. Department of Health and Human Services, Substance Abuse and Mental Health Services Administration (SAMHSA), Office of Applied Studies revealed the following: "In 2006, there were 10.5 million adults aged 18 or older who reported an unmet need for treatment or counseling for mental health problems in the past year. This included 4.8 million adults who did not receive mental health treatment and 5.6 million adults who did receive some type of treatment or counseling for a mental health problem in the past year. Among the 4.8 million adults who reported an unmet need for treatment or counseling for mental health problems and did not receive treatment in the past year, several barriers to treatment were reported. These included an inability to afford treatment (41.5 percent), believing at the time that the problem could be handled without treatment (34.0 percent), not having the time to go for treatment (17.1 percent), and not knowing where to go for services (16.0 percent)." In this book, we hope to address the unmet therapy needs of millions of Americans and help them find competent, caring, and affordable therapists.

If you're reading this book, you are probably looking for (or are already seeing) a psychotherapist. You are also probably fed up with the whole experience—and you have good reason to be. The confusing array of therapist credentials and therapy techniques, as well as conflicting advice from numerous sources, is almost impossible to make sense of, even if you're a professional. It's enough to make you a bit, well, nuts!

It is not an exaggeration to say that today in America we need a therapy revolution. Each year, one in four Americans (that's about 60 million people) ages eighteen and up suffer from minor or major emotional problems, which theoretically should be helped by psychotherapy. But each day, people just like you enter therapy with the belief that they will be helped—and they aren't being helped. In fact, they are being scammed.

When Bad Therapy Happens to Good People

While good therapy can literally be a lifesaver, therapy is not always all it's cracked up to be. In fact, some therapy can actually make people *sicker*. Most people enter therapy hoping to get relief from emotional distress, but many end up unhappier than when they started. You probably know at least one person who has been in (and out of) therapy for years and seems to be getting nowhere. Several therapists and thousands of dollars later, your friend (or you) may find that life seems more empty and painful than ever before. Sadly, this therapy-go-round is considered to be a "normal" state of affairs by many therapists themselves. You will read about some of these experiences in this book—and learn how to avoid them.

What if you are a victim of "hit-and-stay therapy"? That's what we call therapy that just wallops you with an inaccurate or exaggerated diagnosis, and then, session by session, works to reinforce the so-called diagnosis. It keeps you coming back again and again (and opening your wallet, again and again, too). Ineffective therapy methods + uninformed (and vulnerable) patients = therapy dependence, even "therapy addiction." This, too, is part of the therapy crisis.

In *Therapy Revolution*, we will teach you how to prevent—or put a stop to—therapy addiction. You will learn how to spot when a therapist is not giving you your time and money's worth. You will also learn how to recognize and avoid therapists whose therapy practices can actually hook susceptible patients into a never-ending "therapy trap."

Empower Yourself and Demand Accountability

After reading this book you will be able to identify and hire the ethical and *clinically* excellent therapists who deplore these damaging practices. (The word *clinically* is used here to mean relating to psychotherapy) We assure you that good therapists are out there and doing the kind of compassionate and inspirational therapy you may have come to believe doesn't exist. Some therapists, most insurance companies, and many state governments are waking up to the fact that something must be done to ensure that things get better. Serious discussions about setting standards for good therapy are now on the table, and in some states new regulations have even been written.

Unless major *mental illness* (any of the various conditions characterized by impairment of an individual's normal cognitive, emotional, or behavioral functions that can be caused by social, psychological, biochemical, genetic, or other factors such as infection or head trauma), personality disorders, or developmental disorders are the diagnosis, patients like you shouldn't spend too much time or money on therapy, and every good (that is, competent and ethical) therapist knows this. In this book you will learn what questions to ask to ensure that you don't waste years in therapy. You will learn about what to expect during the therapy experience and how to recognize who is and who is not a competent and ethical therapist. You will learn about the centrality of your treatment plan, which is an essential therapy tool. You will learn how to ask your therapist to use a treatment plan if he isn't already doing so.

You will begin to understand your diagnosis and set goals. You will learn about the things you (and your therapist) should do in order to help you reach your goals in a reasonable amount of time. You will also learn how to advocate for yourself during therapy and what to do if you encounter resistance from a therapist. You will learn to insist that your therapist use treatment methods that have been proven to work. You will learn how to recognize when therapy is going nowhere, and when it is time to change therapists or when to seek answers from other disciplines, such as medical or spiritual guidance. You will learn how and why you should demand accountability from your therapist. You will even learn how to tell when therapy has been successful and when it is time for you to move on.

There are many good therapists out there, but there are some who through incompetence or worse are prepared to take your money without getting results, week after week, for years on end. *Therapy Revolution* will help you avoid the bad therapy trap, will help you save money and time, and will give you concrete guidelines you can follow to help make therapy work for you. You will learn how to find *real* help, get better, and move on, so that your life won't be about therapy but about living.

Note to the reader: Throughout this book we use the pronoun "he" for the sake of simplicity, clarity, and consistency. We use it in the spirit of inclusiveness. Similarly, though many choose to use the term "client" or "consumer" to describe those who seek help from psychotherapists, we prefer the term "patient." It seems to us to better describe the more personal relationship a responsible therapist has with those he helps. When the terms "therapy" or "therapist" are used in this book, we are referring to psychotherapy or psychotherapist unless otherwise noted.

Names of patients and therapists, as well as identifying personal and situational details, have been changed to protect the identity of those who have so graciously given us permission to tell their stories.

Chapter 1

WHAT'S IT ALL ABOUT?

Human beings, by changing the inner attitudes of their minds, can change the outer aspects of their lives.

—WILLIAM JAMES

By definition, *psychotherapy* is "The treatment of mental or emotional problems by the use of techniques that are tailored to the unique problems and backgrounds of the individual and that may include talk therapy, behavioral modification, medication, and other treatments." The goal of psychotherapy is to help resolve an individual's mental and emotional problems and, at the same time, teach that individual how to attain the skills needed to deal with life on life's terms.

Therapy is also an inner journey with the therapist as guide. With a good therapist assisting you, your emotions (what you *feel*) begin to get in sync with your intellect (what you *know*). When your head leads and your heart follows, the world becomes an easier, more meaningful place in which to live.

Therapy is not about merely creating an absence of negative feelings or, conversely, about creating happy feelings. It's about helping you live a productive life and about helping you develop and sustain meaningful relationships. It's also about learning and applying the skills you need in order to grow from life's ups and downs.

Downs? "Wait a moment," you might ask, "Why spend all that time and money on therapy if there are still going to be downs when I am through?" Do "ups and downs" mean that sometimes you might be unhappy after finishing therapy? Yes, they do! But with the right therapist you will begin to put your unhappiness in perspective, find ways to grow from the challenges you face, and learn how to create joy in your life. Do "ups and downs" also mean that sometimes, after therapy, you might feel worried or afraid? Yes, again. But with the right kind of therapy, you will be able to put fears and worries in perspective, too. You will even learn that sometimes negative feelings can actually be beneficial—they can help motivate you to change.

If you are experiencing bothersome or even overwhelming negative feelings, or you think that your life stressors are more than you can handle, it might be helpful to speak to a therapist. At the end of this chapter you will find a checklist of symptoms that indicate you might want to consider therapy. Also, you will find a life stressor checklist that can help you determine if you are under a lot of stress right now. This will help you think about how you are coping.

Common Therapy Myths

As a psychotherapist, let me assure you: therapy will not solve all your problems. Don't believe anyone who tells you otherwise—especially a psychotherapist. Solving all life's problems is not even the goal of therapy. What (effective) therapy can do is raise your level of awareness. It can give you the insight and motivation you need to take active steps so you can make good choices in your life. It can also help you make peace with the things you may be unable to change about your life (and yourself).

Have you ever wondered what "going with the flow" really feels like? A skilled therapist can help you recognize when and how to turn your problems into growth opportunities—which might seem like a cliché, until this outlook actually begins to work for you. A skilled therapist will teach you how to do this on your own—to generate a flow of positive outlook in both good times and hard times. *Good therapists are the ones who have the specialized knowledge to actually give you the key to your own transformation.* They also have the sensitivity, training, and ability to work *within* the parameters of your belief system; not aggressively challenging, nor blindly accepting your conditional outlook, but gently helping you deepen your understanding of your life and your life's purpose. They help you resolve to improve.

From our perspective, therapists worth working with have morals and ethics and a respect for their own community and spiritual traditions. Also, it is essential for your therapist to be truly respectful of your spiritual belief system. Additionally, he or she should see psychotherapy as the evolving, imperfect healing system it is—not as an overarching, flawless religion (which some therapists out there believe should replace yours!). A therapist shouldn't be dismissive or impatient of your expressions of belief and shouldn't challenge your deeply held religious convictions.

We recommend that patients actively explore their own religious traditions and think about their spirituality. Polls and studies show that people who are connected to their own traditions are happier with their communities, their families, and their own individual selves. However, a therapist that's right for you should be able to work with you wherever you are on the spectrum of spiritual beliefs, and if not, refer you to someone who is able to do so.

Grady: An Unlikely Eureka

Grady, an engineer in his thirties, had been experiencing anxiety and insomnia for a few months. After serious deliberation, he knew he had to get help. One evening after work he came to see me. I asked him to tell me why he thought he needed psychotherapy. He gripped the arm of the sofa, took a deep breath, and then told me about his mounting anxiety, short temper, and insomnia. He told me about his depression, too, which he (correctly) believed to be caused by fears about losing control. After making a tentative, initial diagnosis of generalized anxiety disorder—which included heart palpitations, insomnia, mood swings, and a growing depression—I asked Grady some questions: "Have you lost someone close to you recently? Have you moved, switched jobs, or experienced another major life change?" His answers were all "no."

Then I asked him about his lifestyle: "Do you exercise regularly? What is your diet like? Have you been using alcohol or other substances?"

"Substances?" asked Grady, "You mean like sleeping pills?"

"Sure. Prescription or nonprescription drugs, even cold medicine can affect your mood. In fact," I told him, "coffee could even be triggering your symptoms. If you drink a lot of it, that is." As soon as I said the word "coffee," Grady had what is called an "Aha Experience." His eyes opened wide and he nodded.

With this brief exchange of simple questions and answers, Grady and I had just uncovered the source of his problems. In this case, Grady's recovery required a "simple fix." He had always been a heavy coffee drinker—drinking four or five cups of freshly ground French roast coffee a day. His workload had increased slightly over the past year, and in order to feel more alert, he began drinking coffee late in the afternoon, which had naturally triggered insomnia. By the morning he was so exhausted from lack of sleep that he would buy a double espresso on the way to work. Soon he was drinking more than ten cups of extremely strong coffee each day.

With instructions to cut down by one cup a day over the next two weeks, then limit himself to one cup of coffee in the morning, Grady left my office a hopeful man. We made one more appointment for a follow-up visit four weeks later so I could be sure there were no additional factors contributing to his problem. Fortunately, though, the case was solved.

Grady's case is the simplest one I've ever had, the one-in-a-million, almost mythical "simple fix." Although during an initial evaluation it is standard for a psychotherapist to ask about substance use, and even specifically mention caffeine, I had never (until that point) had a patient whose problems were caused exclusively by such a one-dimensional trigger as a few cups of coffee. I have also never had such a case since.

The Simple Fix

A *simple fix* is what many patients seek when they enter psychotherapy. Don't be one of them. This simple fix will not happen to you—I personally (almost) guarantee it. What may happen is that when you experience an emotional or mental problem, and you (bravely) decide to seek psychotherapy, you and your therapist may decide that exploring your past could be helpful. If so, you will definitely find that as you expose and discuss your past, life will most emphatically *not* become a bed of thornless roses. Just the opposite will be true at first. Expect to find the experience uncomfortable—even if you believe you are completely prepared to dig deep.

The Exposure Myth

The *exposure myth*, occasionally perpetrated by psychotherapists themselves, is the belief that by exposing a hidden neglect or trauma (usually one that occurred in childhood), or even an external, physical cause (such as extreme stress or substance abuse), all the patient's problems will be solved. Suddenly, the patient's life will become meaningful and happy.

When patients talk about painful events, they are at their most vulnerable. They don't yet know how to build their healed "new" selves because they weren't ready for the confrontation with their unhappy "old" selves. In fact, it is not uncommon to find that patients don't have the emotional scaffolding in place to deal with their pasts. *Emotional scaffolding* is our term for the coping strategies and skills that are taught to a patient by a therapist in order to help the patient manage and deal with the deep inner exploration that may be a part of psychotherapy. These groups of skills act as scaffolding or structures upon which exploration can take place and healthy emotions, feelings, thoughts, and behaviors can be built.

I have seen too many patients who are raw, wounded, and (even after years of therapy), unable to rebuild their lives—they just didn't have the requisite emotional skills in place before they and their therapists plunged in. Psychotherapists who train with me work together with their patients to build the emotional scaffolding they need *before* encouraging their patients to expose painful, deeply private memories. Good therapists know that exposing and discussing everything about their patients' pasts—a common approach, unfortunately—is rarely, if ever, necessary. In some cases untimely or unnecessary exposure to painful recollections may even prevent patients from coping with life at the most basic level. They just shut down. Remember, if you allow a therapist to take you apart, he may not be able to put you back together again.

Good therapists believe in everyone's right to privacy—especially their patients'. They believe it is extremely important to help you understand which parts of your life are relevant and need to be talked about and which areas should remain unexposed. There are some types of therapy, though, that encourage therapists and patients to make an unhealthy breach of boundaries. These methods are a reflection of the culture at large, where privacy and modesty have completely fallen by the wayside.

Nowhere is the lack of respect for boundaries more clearly apparent than in our celebrity culture. There the goal is to attain power and adoration—the kind that comes from gaining the attention of others. In order to get attention, celebrities—and the paparazzi that encourage them—stop at almost nothing.

Although I do practice general psychotherapy, I specialize in anxiety disorders, addiction, co-occurring disorders, and mood disorders, including depression. I have worked with numerous professional athletes, musicians, and other well-known people. Some people, famous and not famous alike, are driven to expose themselves and breach all boundaries, because they are desperate for attention and love. Some will even humiliate themselves to get it. For example, TV reality shows and many talk shows feed upon this neediness. And who hasn't at least glanced at a celebrity tell-all book or magazine in which abusive childhood experiences are described in lurid detail?

Sure, our earliest experiences and relationships influence us greatly. They truly are a very important factor that can help us understand why we are the way we are. All too often though, uncovering and discussing our family's dysfunction (and what family isn't dysfunctional in some way?), has achieved an almost hobbylike status in our culture. We all need to know that talking about our pasts *in and of itself* is not a cure. Exploring the past needlessly, or before one is ready, or exploring it with someone whose trustworthiness is questionable, can be worse than useless. It can cause emotional pain strong enough to instigate a shutdown of feeling and even a shutdown of reason; then the individual's ability to deal with the present, and possibly the future, has been damaged.

Your Emotional Scaffolding: Developing Coping Skills

The systematic, yet personal approach that we know really works (and that differs from other therapeutic approaches), is a combination of the use of proven treatment methods—and the important term here is *proven*—and the therapist's techniques. All effective therapists primarily use proven treatment methods supported by their own studiously developed personal techniques. My personal techniques are based on my own carefully noted observations gleaned from working with thousands of patients over a period of more than twenty-five years. Both the scientific and anecdotal evidence upon which I base my use of methods and techniques support my contention that it is important for your therapist to first help you improve—or, if necessary, develop from scratch—your coping skills and strategies, that is, your emotional scaffolding, *before* digging up and exploring your past.

Your therapist should, beginning from the very first session, evaluate how you cope with problems and challenges. Where your coping skills aren't as strong as they should be, a good therapist will teach you how to strengthen them. Then, and only then, should your therapist ask your permission to go ahead and explore important events in your past.

At some point you may find that even though upon entering therapy you wanted to discuss your past, now you have changed your mind. You may decide that exploring the past isn't important to you right now, or even necessary. Of course, you and your therapist together will have to figure out what is important to discuss, and what is not. However, it should be completely up to you to give the go-ahead. If you feel pressured, bullied, or *very* uncomfortable (remember, at least some level of discomfort is normal in therapy), you should let your therapist know right away. If you do decide to go ahead and discuss your past, you must believe that your therapist is trustworthy. When exploring the past or the present, it should feel as if you are making a journey, with your therapist right there by your side. Sometimes he might be a step or two ahead of you, sometimes a step or two behind, but always there, guiding and supporting you.

As you proceed, if you experience extreme discomfort or unbearable emotional pain, you should feel able to stop the discussion and count on your therapist's full support to do so. You must tell your therapist if you are experiencing extreme discomfort, and he must help you understand and manage that discomfort.

The progressive process outlined above is diametrically opposed to some therapy methods in which the patient is asked shortly after beginning a course of therapy to uncover as many chunks of past information as he or she can, no matter how painful. Don't feel pressured to talk about the past in the first session or two, before your coping strategies and skills have been built and before a trusting relationship between you and your therapist has had some time to develop. Directly ask your therapist to slow down if you feel he is rushing things.

By ripping off the "psychic bandages" that a person has spent years layering on, a hasty therapy technique can cause emotional bleeding that is impossible to stop. *Therapy that pressures the patient to expose too much too soon shows that the therapy process is about achieving the therapist's goals, not the patient's.* Your long-term goals, goals that are in your best interest, should be the focus of therapy. Clearly, therapy should not proceed too slowly or too quickly.

Psychotherapy can and should be about beginning—only when you are truly ready—to uncover, analyze, and rethink influences and choices from your past and, even more important, your present. Your past influences, despite the almost mythical proportions they are given in pop psychology culture, may actually be far less important than you think. My experience shows that it is far too easy to get mired down in the past during therapy and that spending too much time on it is a waste of the patient's time and money. I would rather see a patient work hard to change a disruptive behavior than overanalyze the roots of that behavior. This may not be the most common approach, but it seems to me the most humane one. By exploring an appropriate mix of past influences and present choices with a trustworthy, knowledgeable psychotherapist, you will learn new ways of seeing your life. Then you will be able to apply the emotional skills you have learned in therapy, to *the very next moment in time*—again and again, throughout the moments, days, weeks, and years that make up your life.

When therapy is effective, you will be able to not only cope with events as they are happening or are about to happen, but actually improve your "emotional plans" for your short- and long-term future. And most important, you will be able to apply what you have learned independent of your psychotherapist. You will "graduate," and he or she will no longer be needed.

Your Belief System: The Longer-Shorter Path

If coping skills and strategies are the emotional scaffolding upon which your life reconstruction can begin, your general belief system (of which your spiritual beliefs are an important part) is the foundation upon which your life actually rests. A *dysfunctional belief system* is a set belief or group of beliefs that impair an individual's ability to function in a mentally, emotionally, intellectually, spiritually, and physically healthy manner. A competent therapist can help you smooth out the rough edges of aspects of your foundational belief system. If Grady had come to me professing a belief that chronic use of *opiates* (sedatives that depress the activity of the central nervous system, reduce pain, and induce sleep; with side effects that can include oversedation, nausea, constipation, and death by overdose) would alleviate his anxiety or told me that if he simply quit his job and went on welfare, his tension would dissipate, I would have focused our time together on clarifying these confused beliefs. It is crucial that your therapist have some respect for your spiritual beliefs and the ability to help you strengthen the positive aspects of your general belief system, while helping you steer clear of fallacies.

If Grady had championed irrational beliefs, it would have taken more time than it did to ensure that French roast was indeed his problem. But therapists who are committed to helping patients with their pasts, presents, and futures are the ones who are also committed to ensuring that therapy lasts for a reasonable amount of time. That time frame may be a month, six months, or even a year or more, but *barring a chronic mental illness, personality disorder, late-stage addiction, or other severe problem, if a patient is in therapy for several years, the problem lies with the therapist and not with the patient.*

Of course, sometimes a patient is just not ready to assume intensive responsibility for his or her own life in a shorter time frame. He or she may not want to leave therapy, even though otherwise ready. In this case, much of the therapist's focus should be on helping to motivate the patient to become self-sufficient.

In general, therapists must have the skills necessary to motivate their patients to participate in every important facet of therapy. It is almost never fair for a therapist to say, "The patient doesn't want to change; he's not motivated; there is nothing psychotherapy can do for him." In fact, a therapist must be able to motivate reluctant, recalcitrant, and just plain difficult patients, or send them to a therapist who is able to do so.

It may seem at first glance that learning coping skills, exploring your belief system, and then, if necessary, digging up and exposing your "root problems," past or present, will take much longer than just plunging in right away. However, this is what can be called the "longer-shorter path"; that is, proceeding step-by-(logical)-step, while aiming for a more comprehensive solution. The foundational first steps are:

1. Learning how to cope with the challenges therapy may present by building coping skills and strategies.
2. Refining, strengthening, clarifying, and if truly necessary, modifying your foundational beliefs.
3. Gaining trust in your therapist by developing a relationship with him.

This path, which at first seems lengthy, is in the end far, far shorter indeed. It will prevent repetition of clinical courses of treatment in the long run.

You might wish you were like Grady—able to find peace, happiness, and relief in a cup of decaf. That's because the prospect of therapy—truly effective therapy—can seem daunting. But I want to emphasize (again!) that despite all the hard work psychotherapy entails, it shouldn't (and doesn't) have to take years. In fact, I am very much against therapy taking a long time in most cases. Most people can make inroads into understanding them-selves better and changing their behavior, feelings, and thoughts in a year or less—if their therapist knows how to help them. He must help them learn the requisite coping skills and refine their basic belief system before moving into the realms of exploring the past and, more important, in most cases, the present.

Licensed Professionals: What to Look For

The term "psychotherapist" is an umbrella term for a professional who is licensed to treat patients for mental and emotional problems. "Counselor" is another general term that is used for both licensed professionals and unli-censed nonprofessionals who advise or counsel. A counselor may or may not be a psychotherapist. If you are seeking therapy for emotional problems, mental health issues, addiction, and so on, it is important that you make sure the person you are considering is a licensed psychotherapist. You will most likely be speaking with one or more of the several types of nationally recognized psychotherapists who are licensed by the states in which they work.

Social Workers

Social workers, including licensed clinical social workers (LCSWs, who have taken a detailed state test to prove their competency and have worked thousands of hours under supervision) and licensed masters of social work (LMSWs, who have only taken preliminary competency tests and fulfilled basic requirements) are a popular choice for many people, in large part because their fees are often very reasonable. Social workers used to only do social work, which is about connecting people with the social services they need. Over the years social workers advocated to be able to do the types of counseling work psychotherapists do, too. Today, they are legally allowed to do psychotherapy and counseling, but many still excel at helping connect patients with a variety of social services. Most social workers have received training in clinical skills, so you can feel as confident choosing a social worker as any other type of psychotherapist.

Licensed Marriage and Family Therapists

Licensed marriage and family therapists (LMFTs) are other mental health professionals you might encounter. They are specially trained to help spouses and other family members negotiate the dynamics of their relationships with each other. LMFTs can help you develop skills that can improve your marriage and your relationship with your kids or parents.

Psychologists

Psychologists (Psy.D. or Ph.D.) are nonmedical doctors who are trained to do clinical counseling, including talk therapy and testing. Some also do psychological research. A psychologist can be an excellent choice, though they generally charge more than other nonmedical psychotherapists. This is because their university education has often been costlier and has probably been more extensive. Additionally, in some situations and with the proper education, they may be able to prescribe medication as long as they are supervised by a medical doctor (M.D.). Many insurance companies today are resistant to paying for psychologists and prefer that patients see other types of psychotherapists in order to keep insurance costs lower. Today, the quality of care differential between a psychologist and other psychotherapy professional is not necessarily consequential, so go ahead and choose the type of psychotherapist that appeals to you and fits your budget.

Licensed Mental Health Counselors

Licensed mental health counselors (LMHCs) are becoming extremely popular for a variety of reasons. Each state has its own designated title for mental health counselors, so look under the heading "Mental Health Counselor" or "Professional Counselor" in your state listings. LMHCs are trained and licensed to do the same types of clinical psychotherapy and counseling as psychologists, including talk therapy, testing, and research. Additionally, they are often multicredentialed, which means many of them have special credentials that other psychotherapists don't usually have. These may include but are not limited to:

- Various substance-abuse and addiction specialist credentials, such as *certified alcohol and substance abuse counselor* (CASAC), *certified addiction counselor* (C.A.C.), and so on;
- Education credentials, such as *master of education* (ME.d.), *doctor of education* (Ed.D.);
- Rehabilitation credentials, such as *certified rehabilitation counselor* (C.R.C.), which means they are qualified to help people with social, educational, vocational, and mental problems); and
- Other credentials, including allopathic and alternative medical credentials, such as a *registered nurse* (R.N.) or *credentialed acupuncturist* (C.A.).

Like social workers and psychologists, LMHCs work closely with psychiatrists. Though they aren't able to prescribe medications, many have received education and training in this area. LMHCs generally, though not always, aim for efficacy with the use of solution-oriented, evidence-based therapies, as well as the use of psychoeducation. As mentioned, LMHCs usually have additional certifications, licenses, or degrees. A master's degree or equivalent experience is required for state licensure and rigorous (minimum of two full years) clinical supervision is required before they can become licensed.

Psychiatrists

Psychiatrists are medical doctors who prescribe medication for emotional and mental problems. They may also do research. They usually work hand in hand with other psychotherapy professionals; they may even be part of the same practice. Typically, a psychiatrist sees a patient as needed in order to prescribe or adjust medications. Though some do counseling or talk therapy, most don't.

Psychiatrists like to work closely with nonmedical psychotherapists because it is the licensed mental health counselor, psychologist, or social worker who will have the most in-depth view of a patient and his needs. Most therapists rely on the psychiatrist to ascertain which medication will be right for a patient. An experienced nonmedical psychotherapist, however, may recommend medications for the psychiatrist to prescribe. If an experienced psychotherapist is a specialist in anxiety, for example, he should be up-to-date on anxiety medications and their benefits and drawbacks. He and the psychiatrist can discuss what the best choice is for each particular patient.

As someone who works extensively with patients with mood disorders (including depression), as well as anxiety and addiction, I am always investigating developments in the field, including new medications. When the use of medication is indicated, I may recommend my psychiatric colleagues prescribe specific medications. The psychiatrists I work with will either agree or disagree with my recommendations, and an appropriate course of medication will be decided on, prescribed, and monitored by the psychiatrist with input from the patient and me.

Creative Arts Therapists

There are more types of licensed psychotherapists including *creative arts therapists* (specialists who use various art forms to help achieve psychotherapeutic goals) and others. Check with your state's Education Department or Office of the Professions to find out more about them. If you hear about a therapist who has a credential that is not listed above, also check with your state's registry. Make sure the credential is legitimate, and that your state recognizes and regulates the field.

Pastoral Counselors

Additionally, in most states ordained ministers, priests, and rabbis are legally allowed to do counseling within certain limits. Although many are not licensed professionals, *pastoral counselors* can be helpful in cases where psychological problems are not present but spiritual or moral difficulties are being encountered. Pastoral counselors are ethically obligated to refer people with mental illness or addictions to skilled professionals unless they themselves have had additional training and are licensed to provide care.

Sometimes those with ordination seek degrees in psychology or mental health and can provide well-rounded psychotherapy as well as spiritual guidance. In certain instances, you may want a spiritual advisor and a psychotherapist to work with you concurrently. A bonus to working with a pastoral counselor is that many don't charge for their services—any payment they receive might come from their religious organization, church, synagogue, or mosque.

Psychoanalysts

There are also counselors called *psychoanalysts* who use methods first developed by Sigmund Freud. These methods include techniques designed to help the patient understand his subconscious beliefs, ideas, thoughts, and feelings. Psychoanalysis generally takes several years; we personally know of one individual who was in analysis for twelve years. In New York State a psychoanalyst is a registered professional, but you must check in your state to see if this is the case. If psychoanalysis interests you, check with the American Psychoanalytic Association to make sure the person you are considering has had extensive training.

A Quick Word About Life Coaches

Coaches aim to help people solve various problems, ranging from how to perform successfully during job interviews, to how to better manage confrontations in relationships, to how to define goals and achieve them. Many executives have had good results when working with executive coaches. Also, athletes, dancers, public speakers, pilots, writers, and many other artists and professionals also benefit from working with highly specialized coaches or mentors. However, life coaches aim to coach people about their lives. The difficulty is that one's life is the broadest possible subject—with multiple areas of potential specification.

There are more than three hundred life coach schools and no standardized credentials—anyone can legally call himself a "life coach." We researched coaching schools and found most courses were online, though some required taking some weekend classes in person. There are virtually no academic requirements to enter any life coaching program. The requirements to be able to call yourself a life coach at one of the more highly touted programs was about seventy-five hours of online classes, then you were permitted to use the school's credential. In another famous program, you could begin using their credential as soon as you paid your fee—a fact they heavily advertised. You could "start making money as soon as you register." In other words, there are no standardized life coach requirements or regulations, so use great caution before engaging the services of a coach. Anyone can use *any* credential as a cover for an illicit activity, but it is far easier to do so if there are no regulations concerning a particular field or credential.

However, there are in fact psychotherapists who are also life coaches. They differentiate between the two services they provide, and they feel coaching can really benefit individuals who really don't need psychotherapy, just some focused guidance.

But remember: the majority of life coaches are not psychotherapists, are not allowed to diagnose or practice therapy, and are not recognized as psychotherapists by any medical or psychological counseling association. If you are experiencing mental or emotional problems, we urge you to first get an evaluation from an experienced, well-qualified professional psychotherapist or medical doctor. He or she will be able to help you determine whether or not your problem warrants therapy or whether you should seek advice elsewhere.

The Importance of a Medical Evaluation

Just as some medical doctors aren't in tune with the importance of recommending psychotherapeutic evaluations, some psychotherapists aren't aware of the importance of recommending medical evaluations. Sadly, I would say this is often the case. Illnesses that should be treated medically can sometimes masquerade as emotional problems.

For example, a condition such as *mitral valve prolapse* (a common disorder where the valve between the heart's left upper chamber and the left lower chamber doesn't close properly) can cause symptoms of anxiety, including heart palpitations. *Hypothyroidism* (an underactive thyroid gland) can cause depression and irritability, and there are numerous other medical conditions that can cause psychological symptoms. Additionally, medications themselves can cause psychological symptoms, including medications given to alleviate psychological problems!

It is important that the psychotherapist you choose to hire works well with your psychiatrist or other medical doctor, if you have one. Your psychotherapist is the caregiver who will spend the most time getting to know you. He or she will be able to advocate for you and even ask your other doctor to prescribe appropriate medications if he agrees that you need them. For this reason, if medication is necessary, it is important that your therapist be someone with an up-to-date knowledge of medications—he doesn't have to be a doctor, but he should keep abreast of the latest drug therapies, something many counselors, especially those who work in addiction therapy, do.

Connie: Incorrectly Prescribing Medications

Connie, a forty-year-old petite mother of two from Manhattan's Upper West Side, is a psychologist herself. She was referred to me by her rabbi. She saw me individually and occasionally also with her husband. She had been diagnosed by her former psychotherapist as having anxiety disorder and major depression.

She told me that her previous experience with talk therapy seemed to be getting her nowhere, so she decided to see a medical doctor. He prescribed Valium (a benzodiazepine—a class of drugs that act as tranquilizers and that are commonly used in the treatment of anxiety) and a sleep aid called Ambien (a sedative-hypnotic, or sedative medication that depresses the activity of the central nervous system, reduces anxiety, and induces sleep). Both are addictive medications generally prescribed for anxiety and insomnia, though both of these types of medications are known for exacerbating depression. Also, it is generally undesirable to prescribe addictive medications right away; if possible, every other reasonable and effective non-narcotic option should be tried first.

Both these medications were obviously contributing to Connie's deepening depression and chronic fatigue. She was practically in a stupor when she first came to see me—that is, in a pharmacologically induced blindfold, unable to perceive or think about her life at all. She was numb. All she knew was that she needed help. I sent Connie to a psychiatrist I work with regularly. Then he and I discussed her case, and I suggested that he immediately begin to titrate—slowly reduce or increase a medication to avoid withdrawal symptoms or uncomfortable/dangerous side effects (in this case, wean her off the Valium)— which he agreed to do at once. Then he decided to introduce two nonaddictive, antianxiety medications that would work symbiotically to alleviate her symptoms. Next, he titrated her off the Ambien.

In Connie's case, prescribed medicines had not been prescribed correctly. They were not only producing an extreme sedative effect, they were causing a host of painful and dangerous physical side effects, including kidney problems and gastritis. Surprisingly, her doctor never monitored her for these not-uncommon problems. Within weeks of being put on appropriate, nonaddictive medications at the correct dosages, Connie's symptoms abated, and she began to make some inroads in her marriage and her life in general.

In an ideal world, all anxiety disorders would respond to deep breathing, guided visualizations, and simple behavioral modification; indeed, whenever possible, I try these methods alongside proven techniques. But anxiety, depression, and other disorders can cause such extreme suffering that almost every minute of a person's life can seem unbearable. Sometimes, treating and relieving the symptoms medically is the first step. Then therapy can begin. In psychotherapy, the judicious use of medication can help a patient (who is comfortable with the idea of taking medication) make gains so that he or she is not distracted by painful symptoms.

When Should I Consider Therapy?

✓ Symptom Checklist

If you have frequent and/or ongoing instances of any of the following, you should get an evaluation from a skilled psychotherapist. He may also refer you to a medical doctor, if indicated. If you suspect a medical condition is causing your symptoms, then get an evaluation from a psychiatrist or other medical doctor first.

- ❏ Sadness/depression (the "blues")
- ❏ Any overwhelming or ongoing fear
- ❏ Anxiety/extreme tension
- ❏ Nervousness
- ❏ Hysteria
- ❏ Memory problems
- ❏ Overwhelming guilt
- ❏ Scattered or confused thinking
- ❏ Overwhelming suspiciousness or hostility
- ❏ Strange or bizarre thoughts
- ❏ Anger/impulse control (you become easily upset and lash out verbally or physically)
- ❏ Identity problems (questions about sexuality, what is the meaning of [my] life, confusion about long-term goals, career choices, group loyalties, friendships)
- ❏ Spirituality problems (moral, religious, and spiritual questions and issues, cult membership, etc.)

✓ Life Stress Checklist

If you believe that any of the following life stressors are causing any of the symptoms from the Symptom Checklist (or other related or unusual symptoms), you may want to see a psychotherapist. If you are feeling that you are in crisis and have thoughts of harming yourself or others, you should call 911 or go to the nearest emergency room and notify a trusted friend or family member.

- ❑ Death of a family member
- ❑ Divorce
- ❑ Marriage (yes, even the good things in life cause stress)
- ❑ Terminal illness (one's own or that of a family member)
- ❑ Physical incapacitation, chronic pain, or chronic illness
- ❑ Drug or alcohol abuse by self or family member
- ❑ Mental illness of self or family member
- ❑ Loss of job or job change
- ❑ Moving house
- ❑ Change of school (for children, but can be adults too)
- ❑ Relationship/relational problems (unable to get along with spouse, family, friends, coworkers)
- ❑ Academic problems (poor grades, inability to retain information, problems with teachers, deadlines)
- ❑ Occupational problems (lateness, absences, problems with boss, coworkers)
- ❑ Victim of abuse
- ❑ Victim of crime
- ❑ Criminal/abusive actions of self or family member
- ❑ Extreme loneliness/lack of community membership or friendships

Chapter 2

The Successful Therapy Formula

Before anything else, preparation is the key to success.

—Alexander Graham Bell

Successful therapy, that is, therapy that effectively changes how you live your life, must contain five fundamental ingredients:

1. The therapist must be a motivated, experienced professional.
2. The therapist must use evidence-based treatments; that is, proven methods and techniques.
3. Therapy must be carried out in a reasonable treatment time frame.
4. The therapist's per-hour fee and the entire cost of the course of treatment must be fair and reasonable.
5. The patient must be a motivated patient.

It is important to know that while all the above ingredients must be present, they can be present in varying proportions. So, you may decide that a therapist who costs a bit more than average, but who is highly motivated and experienced, might be a better choice for you than a therapist who costs less but doesn't have as much experience, or vice versa. It is also important to note that just because a therapist charges more doesn't necessarily mean that he is a better therapist. However, therapists with more experience sometimes do tend to charge more (though not always).

Ingredient No. 1:
Motivated, Experienced Professional

A therapist must be *motivated*—that means he must really believe in what he's doing and be willing to work hard to help his patients reach their goals. Your therapist must have faith that the techniques and methods he chooses to use will produce a successful outcome. You may sense, consciously or subconsciously, whether or not your therapist feels good about these choices. You may also sense whether your therapist believes you are making progress—however, you should rely on more than just your gut feeling. Throughout this book we will teach you what questions to ask your therapist and how to ask them in order to really gauge whether or not therapy is working for you.

If your therapist is confident in his skills and abilities, he will give you the confidence you need to move forward. His job is, in part, to inspire you to believe in the possibility of positive change, and, of course, to help you make that change happen. It's simple: if he's a believer, you'll be a believer, too; if he works really hard, you most likely will as well.

But motivation isn't enough. Plenty of hucksters throughout history have had mountains of motivation. They've been extremely motivated to sell those bottles of snake oil, Kabbalah water, or antiwrinkle cream (guaranteed to change your life, of course). And some of these guys even believe in what they are doing. But they lack the three essential qualities that denote the difference between a dedicated professional and a motivated quack: education, training, and experience.

An experienced therapist should have at least a few, if not several, years of education, and plenty of supervised, on-the-job training. He should be someone who has honed his therapy skills under supervision and is now able to employ a variety of methods as indicated by his patients' needs. He should have a repertoire of at least a few techniques that he is very comfortable using. These techniques should be nearly second nature to him. He should wield them like "the force." He should also have the experience to know which techniques will work with which patient, since not all patients respond to the same clinical methods.

Staying Current

An experienced therapist should keep improving—his education shouldn't end when he graduates from college. He should be aware of the current discoveries in the field. Psychotherapy, like all fields, improves regularly. Just as you (hopefully) wouldn't schedule surgery with a heart surgeon who hasn't cracked a book or attended a seminar since graduating medical school thirty years ago, you wouldn't schedule a therapy session with a therapist who last studied under Sigmund Freud.

Therapists should be constantly upgrading their education by attending seminars where they learn about the latest proven techniques. They should also polish the techniques they already know. They should subscribe to professional journals and read as much as possible in order to keep abreast of new discoveries, including improvements in medication. They should not only be up-to-date on treatment methods, but they should also be up-to-date on ethics and the business of running their practice. An experienced therapist who cares about his work will be happy to tell you which educational programs, seminars, and conferences he has recently attended. He might have even written articles in newspapers, magazines, or professional journals—you can ask him to give you a copy or two to take home and read.

A Broad and Diverse Practice

An experienced therapist will also be one who has a broad worldview and who has worked with a variety of types of patients. Why is this essential? Doesn't it make sense to choose a therapist who has worked exclusively with patients just like you? The surprising answer is "no"! Therapists need a broad range of experiences because patients rarely fit into one category. A museum curator living in Philadelphia who has anxiety and abuses alcohol may, oddly enough, have more in common with a farmer from Idaho who abuses alcohol than other anxious museum curators who live on the East Coast. There is always some overlap in outlook, behavior, and symptoms with patients from seemingly disparate backgrounds.

When a therapist has had a broad range of experiences with many types of patients (those who have many different reasons for seeking therapy), he will develop a broader range of techniques and a better understanding of psychotherapy than someone who has only worked with one type of patient. The truism about travel broadening and enriching a person can be applied to the therapy experience as well. A "well-traveled" therapist—one who has had a variety of therapeutic experiences—is able to see potential for effective therapy to take place where therapists with less diverse training can't. He will most likely have a deeper understanding of life and of human nature in general and therapy is, in essence, about these amorphous subjects. He will also be able to intuit which therapy methods should be used and adapt them as needed—even when confronting problems he may not have encountered before. A well-traveled therapist makes for well-rounded therapy, and he will be the kind of therapist who will be able to help his patients draw on all their own life experiences to positively effect change. After he has gained broad experience, he might choose to specialize in one or two areas.

Ingredient No. 2:
Evidence-based Treatments

Evidence-based treatments is just a fancy term for *proven* treatment methods or techniques. It is so important that your therapist, like your dentist, mechanic, or hairdresser, uses methods that have been proven to work. Studies done by universities and research institutes show that some types of therapy treatment methods currently in use work and some don't. Many states are beginning to require psychotherapists to use proven treatment methods.

If our dentist, who we happen to like and respect, told us to brush our teeth with chopped liver, we might comply since we generally trust him to take excellent care of our dental health. We would be disappointed and prob-ably annoyed to learn, however, that brushing teeth with chopped liver is not only a colossal waste of money, but completely ineffective in the fight against cavities. Not one study (that we know of) shows that chopped liver has anti-cavity properties. Your therapist should also not use *chopped liver therapy*, that is, therapy methods that have not been proven to work.

Modern psychotherapy as we know it is a comparatively young healing discipline and it seems to have put forth more than its share of extravagantly foolish techniques. Occasionally, these have been posited by those seeking to shake up the system or make names for themselves, rather than to create healing results. Over time, most of these techniques have been discarded and forgotten, but it seems that some of them crop up in different guises again and again. Some of these methods are merely useless, but a few can actually cause harm. Of course, for every thousand professionals who say a method is non-sense, you will find one who swears by it. In general, I recommend you lis-ten to the thousand rather than the one.

An example of one of these chopped liver therapy methods that has almost global name recognition is *primal scream therapy*—the stuff of all-time great rock band names, certainly. You might be most familiar with its signa-ture technique: the primal scream. The primal scream, where patients and their therapists simply scream, may be good fun, but it's not good therapy. Most therapists have debunked the value of the primal scream. Most of the literature that mentions it says that this method demonstrates no therapeu-tic results whatsoever. It's not hard to imagine why, since no scientific stud-ies have been done that prove otherwise. Yet, even today, a handful of therapists still employ primal scream therapy.

Another technique that is popular, but one that I am strongly against using, is called *flooding*. This technique bombards, or floods, the patient with negative stimuli related to a trauma that he has endured. Occasionally, inex-perienced therapists like to use this aggressive technique because it has been touted as an easy way to get results—fast. However, the results are usually the retraumatization of the patient. This technique primarily causes needless suffering, something all ethical therapists are against.

In addition to using useless or harmful techniques, a therapist might use a proven technique in the wrong situation. There are many techniques that are proven to work *only* with specific problems. Sometimes these might be overenthusiastically employed by therapists who have had some success with these techniques and think they have now found a panacea.

For example, there is a technique called systematic desensitization that works very well in many instances. It helps reduce anxiety and can even help people overcome phobias. How it works is simple. The therapist sets up a series of situations, each one progressively more anxiety-provoking than the next, so that the patient learns to cope with his fears step-by-step. A patient who is afraid to fly may first be driven by an airport. Then he'll visit the airport. In the next step he will sit on a plane on a runway. Then he will spend some time on a taxiing plane. All the while he is becoming desensitized to the stimuli that trigger his fears. At some point he will hopefully be ready to fly. There have been many studies that show systematic desensitization is extremely effective when used in this manner.

However, *systematic desensitization* does not work at all with people who are out of touch with reality, such as those with schizophrenia. Nor is it helpful for people who have experienced physical and/or sexual abuse. Unfortunately, some therapists try to apply this technique across the board. More experienced professionals then have to pick up the pieces. It is extremely important that the evidence-based treatment method used is appropriate for the patient's situation.

Therapists who use the *confrontation technique*—an unproven technique in which a psychotherapist forcefully confronts a patient with a traumatic event or harsh reality or criticism in order to "attack and shatter" the patient—believe that it can bring about an immediate realization and radical, positive change to the patient's psyche. Most therapists agree that this technique can be extremely painful and harmful, and it has limited use. Perhaps in some restricted use it can be effective. I am sorry to say that most often it is used very inappropriately, as in the case of Angela.

Angela: Misusing Therapeutic Techniques

A twenty-five-year-old patient of mine, Angela, was studying to be a real estate agent. She was having a hard time focusing both at work and at home because she was experiencing severe mood swings linked, in large part, to a long-term history of being physically abused.

Angela had been regularly and forcefully confronted by her previous therapist. He told her that she would never get better no matter what kind of therapy she tried. He said, "Based on your history of not succeeding at therapy, your situation is hopeless." Now, in rare cases, with the right kind of patient and with the right timing and context, a variant of this technique can certainly be motivating. In certain situations, a variant I call compare and contrast therapy *can help create enough energy in the patient to stimulate momentum for change. This is a modified confrontation technique I use in which I gently confront a patient with an alternate point of view or other information and encourage the patient to actively compare and contrast the information presented to him, with his previous understanding. This may involve gently confronting the patient with challenging information in order to help bring about change. Unlike the confrontation technique, compare and contrast therapy is used very briefly, in very small, manageable bites at junctures where the potential for change is the greatest.*

However, for Angela, a traumatized patient with mood swings, the use of forceful confrontation only devastated her emotionally. We spent several sessions devoted to "decontaminating" the effects of her previous destructive, painful encounters.

Checking Up on Proven Treatments

So how do you know if the techniques a therapist is using have been proven effective? First, ask the therapist if he uses evidence-based techniques. Don't be afraid to put this question to him directly. It also can't hurt that he knows you are educated enough to ask.

Next, familiarize yourself a bit with the most commonly accepted evidence-based techniques. Some techniques or styles of therapy that have been scientifically proven to be safe and effective in a broad variety of cases include:

- *Cognitive behavioral therapy* (CBT): a relatively short-term form of psychotherapy based on the concept that the way we think about things affects how we feel emotionally. CBT focuses on thinking, behavior, and communication in the present rather than past experiences and is oriented more toward problem solving than some other kinds of psychotherapy. CBT has been proven to be highly effective with many types of patients.
- *Motivational interviewing*: a technique used in psychotherapy in which the psychotherapist helps the patient explore and resolve ambivalence about troubling issues, thereby helping him become motivated to make behavioral changes. Motivational interviewing has been proven to be highly effective with many types of patients.
- *Rational emotive therapy*: a form of cognitive behavioral therapy that helps patients understand that their beliefs about adversity contribute to their experience of adversity. This rational therapeutic technique has repeatedly been proven to be effective for many types of patients.
- *Cognitive restructuring*: a technique that helps an individual replace irrational, distorted beliefs, with beliefs that are more factual, and therefore, beneficial. Cognitive restructuring is a proven technique.
- *Brief psychotherapy*: short-term psychotherapy generally recommended in order to help patients quickly overcome major situational problems

by focusing on solutions to these problems, rather than by addressing deep underlying personality issues, though some practitioners do use this form of therapy for a variety of serious problems. Today there is disagreement about various approaches of brief psychotherapy, so be sure to ask a therapist who uses this style of therapy to clarify what the term means as he sees it.

- *Dialectical behavior therapy*: the first type of therapy proven effective in the treatment of patients with personality disorders, it is based in part on cognitive behavioral therapy as well as other techniques, including the development of mindfulness/awareness, emotional regulation, and more.

There are many more, but this list includes some of the foundational ones. Each of these techniques is not right to use in every case, but they have at least been rigorously studied using real-life patients and therapists. Again, you should feel free to ask your therapist what kinds of techniques he uses, and also about his training and experience with these techniques. Where and when did he learn how to use the technique? How long has he been using it to treat patients? That way you can be sure he is not only using methods that work, but that he is using them appropriately.

It is not urgent that you understand every detail of the techniques your therapist will be using to help you; you just need to know that the techniques are proven to work and that your therapist has solid experience working with them. What is essential is that you have a *general* understanding of how your therapist plans to help you.

In Chapter 3, and in other places in this book, we will show you what kinds of questions to ask your therapist about his clinical methods and what kind of response you should get. We will give you a detailed plan to help you get the most effective therapy possible.

Ingredient No. 3:
Reasonable Treatment Time Frame

A *treatment time frame* is the period of time treatment will take and which should take into account and include the frequency of therapy sessions. When I was a clinical supervisor in charge of a program for mentally ill chemical abusers, I was part of a committee that put together a "treatment-structure standards manual," used by a broad range of clinicians. This is a rather complicated title for a manual that simply describes how psychotherapy patients should, ideally, be treated. This particular manual included, among other things, what we called a "threshold" for the number of patient visits. This means that our committee did our best to set standards for the minimum and maximum number of visits needed in order to treat patients effectively, ideally in the shortest possible period of time.

With the health maintenance organization (HMO) explosion in the 1970s and 1980s, medical and psychology professionals had to prove to insurance providers that they weren't wasting their reimbursement money. Many insurance companies began to limit the number of annual mental health and substance abuse visits they were willing to pay for. Today that number is on average about twenty visits per year for mental health and forty to sixty for substance abuse. It is important to check with your insurance company before you begin therapy if you plan on relying on insurance coverage to pay for it. You must be vigilant—treat your insurance benefits as if they were your own money in your personal "bank" account. Watch and make sure that your therapist is billing the insurance company correctly; also watch and make sure that the insurance company is giving you all the care you are entitled to receive.

On the plus side of these restrictions, by limiting the number of visits allowed, many professionals have been forced to carefully evaluate what treatments they recommend. Many are less likely to waste insurance dollars by recommending useless treatments. On the down side, insured patients who don't fit the general mold might have a hard time getting the special care they need—unless they pay for it out of pocket.

Additionally, unscrupulous therapists might schedule a patient for the maximum number of annual visits covered by insurance, whether or not the patient needs them. This is why the use of a detailed, written treatment plan with clearly defined goals and objectives and an approximate time frame for treatment should be used in any course of therapy. You will learn more about the importance of the treatment plan in Chapter 5.

Today we are experiencing the repercussions of the development of treatment standards as directed by HMOs. The difficulties involved in managing the insurance side of their practices means that expenses for psychotherapists have skyrocketed. Though hospitals and clinics almost always take insurance, today most therapists in private practice don't. (Note: if a therapist does agree to accept your insurance, then he cannot legally ask you for additional money if a session runs over the scheduled time.)

Another repercussion of the insurance crunch is that some therapists who take insurance have responded by recommending courses of treatment they know insurance companies automatically approve, whether the patient needs them or not. That would be like a medical doctor giving you an appendectomy for an ingrown toenail. Fortunately, the vast majority of insurance companies will ask the therapist to fax a copy of the treatment plan to them so they can verify that the course of treatment is one that is generally recommended. Of course, ethical therapists are working harder and more efficiently than ever to deliver effective treatment to their patients now that insurance companies limit the number of visits.

Alistair: When a Realistic Treatment Time Frame Isn't Established

Alistair, one of my patients, is a forty-five-year-old city adminis-trator with a great sense of humor and a real knack for helping to make his city one of the most livable in the country. He had a long history (twenty years) of mild depression and anxiety. For three years he was in treatment with a psychologist I will call Dr. Parks. Dr. Parks used a technique called insight-oriented therapy, which is an approach that helps the patient understand himself and his motivations. This tech-nique is safe and generally quite effective.

Unfortunately, the doctor never asked Alistair some fundamental questions about his life beforehand, and therefore never found out about Alistair's history of abusing alcohol and sleeping pills. Oops. Because of his egregious error, Dr. Parks treated Alistair for depression and anxiety, ignoring his undiscovered addiction to alcohol and sleep-ing pills. He even sent Alistair to a psychiatrist who, on his advice, prescribed antidepressants. These medications were deactivated by Alis-tair's alcohol and sleeping pill consumption and were rendered useless (though very expensive). Alistair, who was ashamed of his drinking, never at any point volunteered information about his substance abuse. He sheepishly told me, "Well, if Dr. Parks would have asked me, I would have told him. But he never did ask."

So Alistair ended up wasting three years in therapy. Even without full knowledge of Alistair's condition, Dr. Parks, an experienced psy-chologist, knew that the treatment time for mild depression could have taken as little as six months to one year. Certainly, there should have been some improvement during that time frame. Because the doctor never discussed treatment time frames with his patient, Alistair kept coming in to see him, despite getting nowhere, week after week, year after year. Alistair is bright and well educated, but he had no idea what to expect from therapy, and therefore no real way of knowing that his therapy was going down the tubes. Finally, a family member suggested he find another therapist. He scheduled an initial evaluation with me.

After thoroughly evaluating Alistair, and finding out, during the first session, about his abuse of alcohol and sleeping pills, I immediately scheduled him to see his psychiatrist for an update in his medication. I recommended an antidepressant and antianxiety and anticraving medications, which the psychiatrist agreed to prescribe. Alistair also began seeing me for psychotherapy. In addition, I recommended he attend group therapy twice a week. In our one-on-one sessions, I primarily used motivational interviewing. Alistair's medicine levels were regularly monitored and adjusted, and he voluntarily submitted to Breathalyzers. At the end of three months he was able to remain completely abstinent from all substances, and his depression and anxiety had lifted. Together, we began to work even harder on developing skills that would help him understand and regulate his moods and symptoms. He began to learn how to develop mastery of his emotions, thoughts, and behaviors.

Now, three months and one week after his initial visit, Alistair feels substantially better. He is still going to group therapy once a week (and going with his wife and children for family therapy twice a month), but I estimate that within a three- to four-month treatment time frame, he will be able to leave therapy for good. When I asked for his permission to include his story in this book, he told me, with tears in his eyes, "Nobody has ever been able to help me before. You and the psychiatrist really knew exactly what to do to help me, and you just got on with it. You helped me do the hard work I needed to do in record time. You didn't drag therapy out."

This experience is not unique—most patients are happy and grateful when therapy has been effective and their suffering has ended. This scenario plays out many times every day as people find help through psychotherapy. I find that patients are the most grateful when they receive *realistic* information at the outset of therapy and pleased when goals are set and a positive outcome has finally been achieved.

What Is a Realistic Treatment Time?

You can take advantage of the general recommendations for treatment protocols. If you have received a diagnosis, ask your therapist what the *standard, recommended* treatment time frame is for your particular problem. A reasonable response may be, "It depends on how well you do," but still, you are entitled to know the general time frame and protocols based on insurance company guidelines. Also, your therapist will probably refer to the *Diagnostic and Statistical Manual of Mental Disorders* (DSM-IV-TR) in order to clarify your diagnosis and help develop your treatment protocol. If you don't have a specific diagnosis such as *major depression* (a mental illness that affects a person's mood, thoughts, and activity level and often involves feelings of profound sadness), anxiety, or schizophrenia, you can still ask your therapist what is generally recommended for people with problems like yours.

It is important for you to believe that the treatment time frame your therapist recommends is reasonable. A 2008 study published in the British journal *Psychology and Psychotherapy: Theory, Research and Practice* showed that only 40 percent of patients who had recently left psychotherapy felt that the therapy ended at the appropriate time, 37 percent felt that it had ended earlier than it should have, and 23 percent felt that the therapy went on for too long. Did these patients have a treatment time frame in their treatment plans? Possibly not.

Your therapist should regularly check in with you as you progress and discuss whether or not the time frame for the completion of therapy will be as expected. When combined with the use of appropriate methods, setting up realistic treatment time frames means that therapy has a better chance of succeeding.

Don't be afraid to ask your therapist directly, "How long do you expect treatment for my problem to take?" He should be willing to explain how long (approximately) treatment should take. He should be able to estimate a reasonable treatment time frame: a beginning, middle, and end of your psychotherapy experience. It should be a time frame you are comfortable with on an emotional level. *It should also be a time frame you are comfortable with financially*. Throughout this book you will learn how to maximize the value you get for the money you spend on therapy.

Ingredient No. 4: Fair and Reasonable Cost

Assuming that you are paying out of pocket—which is often the case when seeing a psychotherapist in private practice—affordability may be foremost in your mind. A fair and reasonable cost is one that takes into account: (1) the therapist's education and training, including ongoing coursework, which must be regularly updated to recertify psychotherapists in some specialties; and (2) the experience of the therapist and location of his practice. A very experienced therapist based in Biloxi, Mississippi, may charge less for a session than a relatively inexperienced therapist based in Los Angeles, California. Location is certainly one of the more influential factors in determining cost.

Unfortunately for patients, there is no official table of therapist rate guidelines. However, there are some resources that can help you get a better idea of what a fair cost will be for therapy sessions in your area. Local

chapters of national professional associations such as the American Psychiatric Association, the American Mental Health Counselors Association,
the American Psychological Association, and the National Association of
Social Workers can help. A list of professional associations you can contact
can be found in the "Resources" at the end of this book.

Generally speaking, a visit to a psychotherapist in a government-funded
clinic can cost anywhere from five to fifty dollars. A visit to a psychotherapist in private practice can generally cost anywhere from eighty to five hundred dollars depending on the professional's education, experience, and
location. One important thing to keep in mind: a fair cost goes hand in hand
with a realistic treatment time frame. A therapist must be upfront about the
(approximate) number of visits he thinks you will need to achieve your goals,
how often these visits will be scheduled, and how much each visit will cost.
Many therapists have sliding rate scales based on income; in Chapter 3 we
will show you how to ask your therapist about his fees and negotiate an
affordable rate if finances are a serious impediment to getting help. We will
also show you which questions to ask to ensure that the end of a course of
therapy happens sooner rather than later.

Ingredient No. 5: Motivated Patient

It may seem that the patient's own motivation would be exclusively under
the patient's locus of control, but that is not the case. Yes, of course you *should*
be motivated to work hard in therapy, and you should ideally arrive at your
sessions ready to do whatever it takes to progress. But your therapist must
partner with you in this area. He should work right alongside you to enhance
your motivation levels. He can do this in a few ways.

First, he must create a trusting alliance with you. By creating an environment where you feel comfortable expressing your feelings on any subject,
including the therapy process itself, a therapist will be able to assist you in
developing the inner impetus you need to get better and move on. Open
conversations where your therapist makes every attempt to support you can
inspire you to trust him and therefore work harder.

Next, by helping you set realistic goals and by establishing a reasonable time frame in which to accomplish those goals, your therapist will help fuel your motivation. He should encourage you to ask questions and develop a good understanding of what the therapeutic experience will be like. He should present a realistic idea of what therapy can accomplish for you. *Expectations grounded in reality are essential to success in therapy.* If you are given unrealistic expectations, the kind that any therapy will naturally fail to meet, your motivation can grind to a halt.

Additionally, right at the outset, your therapist will probably mention that he will have fairly regular "check-ins" with you. Even if he doesn't mention them, a good therapist will steer some session time that way. During these check-ins, you will pause from discussing other issues and instead discuss how you are feeling about the therapy experience itself. Like having your oil checked and changed, your tires rotated, and your gas tank filled, these brief check-in discussions operate as psychotherapy pit stops. You and your therapist will use these talks to determine if you are fully capable of proceeding, and that you are "fueled up" and ready to complete the next lap. During these talks your therapist will make every attempt to both bolster and assess your motivation levels. Sometimes merely reminding you of the importance of your input is enough to get you fired up and ready to work.

I specialize in a few areas of treatment, one of which is the treatment of *anxiety disorders*. An anxiety disorder is a chronic condition characterized by excessive and persistent apprehension with physical symptoms such as sweating, palpitations, and feelings of nervousness. Patients experiencing anxiety are usually extremely motivated to feel better and to make therapy work. I see many patients with anxiety. Because their motivation levels can be quite high, my need to focus on motivating them is often minimal.

I am also, however, an addiction specialist. One type of program I have directed over the years treats patients who are not only substance abusers, but are also mentally ill. These patients are, as a rule, extremely unmotivated— at least when they first show up for treatment. Many of them do not want to be in therapy, and they are angry at me, my staff, and the world.

Gerry: Resistant to Change

Gerry was a successful financial whiz kid. Originally from Philadelphia's wealthy Main Line, he got his M.B.A. from a prestigious Ivy League university. By the time he was twenty-four, he had made more than $15 million as a futures trader. He thrived on excitement. He had a fantastic loft in lower Manhattan with wraparound views, a beautiful, accomplished girlfriend, and all the "toys" a man with his money could buy. He appeared to be heading only for more success.

Gerry was rarely, if ever, down about anything. Why should he be? Life was looking good. In fact, Gerry was always upbeat—too upbeat. To take some of the edge off his natural highs, he began drinking. To fight his after-drinking blues, he began using cocaine. Soon, his life spiraled out of control. Eight months after he began using drugs, he was arrested for driving while intoxicated and was mandated by the courts to get treatment. He arrived at my program with a chip the size of the futures' market on his shoulder.

Because Gerry was suffering from **mania** *for days at a time, he didn't feel he had a problem. Mania is recognized by extremely hyperactive (and often over-elated or enthusiastic) thoughts, moods, and/or behaviors that can be caused by the presence of a mental illness such as bipolar disorder or substance abuse. Mania can cause aggression, lead to other dangerous behaviors that can hurt the self and others, and can even lead to a break with reality. This denial in and of itself was a large part of Gerry's problem. Fortunately we were able to diagnose his problem almost immediately. We got him on the right medication* *and within two months his mood stabilized. We also immediately began treating him for his addiction and began giving him psychotherapy. To say he was resistant is an understatement. He showed up for the program only because if he didn't, he would be in violation of a court order. Even though he lost his girlfriend, friends, and job because of his illness and addiction, he had no desire to change. He groaned, complained, and cursed his way through the first weeks of therapy. Mania—and drugs and alcohol—felt too good to give up.*

Little by little, we worked on getting Gerry to want to change. We asked pointed questions about the consequences of his out-of-control behavior and got him to really slow down and examine the issues in his life. We also asked him how he envisioned his future, and how he expected to achieve this vision. His illness had prevented him from even thinking beyond tomorrow, but in therapy he began to make long-term goals and plans—for the first time since leaving college.

Today, Gerry is doing great. He has gone back to grad school and this time, he is working on a degree in veterinary medicine. He loves animals and wants to be in an environment that will not trigger his disastrous highs. He invested what remained of his money and used the gains to pay for his education. He also donated a substantial amount to a mental health research program. Because the therapists he worked with unlocked the key to his inner motivation, today Gerry is well adjusted, in control of his life, and working hard to achieve his goals.

My staff knows that it is up to *us* to motivate these patients. We operate under the premise that there are rarely, if ever, excuses for not helping patients get motivated. We do the hard work it takes to find out what methods can help these patients *want* to get better. Have we ever had patients who were extremely resistant? Sure. But those patients taught us even more about how to motivate even the most recalcitrant. Psychotherapists who work with mentally ill substance abusers, those who have what is called *co-occurring disorders* (in this usage, two or more illnesses or disorders that occur simultaneously and may be interactive; frequently used to describe the simultaneous occurrence of a mental illness and an addiction), are experts at helping patients tap into their deepest selves to find the sources of healthy inspiration and motivation.

Checklist for Success

Remember:

1. The therapist must be a motivated, experienced professional.
2. The therapist must use evidence-based methods (proven methods and techniques).
3. Therapy must be carried out in a reasonable time frame.
4. There must be a fair and reasonable cost.
5. The patient must be a motivated patient—that's you!

How can you find out, without spending months in therapy, if a therapist has the five foundational ingredients necessary to giving good therapy? By asking questions and listening closely to the answers. Also, you will probably need to observe the therapist over the course of a couple of sessions. In Chapters 3 and 4, you will find out which questions to ask and how to ask them. You will also learn how to evaluate the answers. You will be given the tools you need to find out if the essentials, and more, are there.

Chapter 3

Don't Hire a Therapist . . . Until You Make This Phone Call

A good decision is based on knowledge and not on numbers.

—Plato

I've got nothing against blind dates. In fact, I know of a successful marriage or two that resulted from these much-castigated experiences. But setting up a blind date, or "blind appointment," with a therapist is not something I would ever recommend. Since an initial therapy session, which generally includes a preliminary evaluation, can cost anywhere from $150–500 or more with a therapist in private practice, it's a good idea to do a brief phone interview before scheduling your first appointment. Remember—when you hire any service provider you want him to (1) be qualified to do the job and (2) be someone you feel comfortable working with. A therapist should be able to convince you he fits the bill on both counts—preferably before you meet.

Another reason I recommend you do a phone interview is that it will be far easier for you to say "no" to a therapist on the phone than in person. When a person meets a therapist face-to-face, he can be more easily convinced to begin a course of therapy. Needless to say, it will be much more difficult for you to extricate yourself from therapy that isn't going anywhere than to say "this isn't right for me" in the first place (preferably over the phone).

Most people feel uncomfortable rejecting someone. It is not uncommon for a patient to decide to end a course of therapy, then spend several sessions (and several hundred dollars) working up the "guts" to tell the therapist of his decision. Remember—you don't owe your therapist an apology if working with him isn't right for you. But by minimizing the risk of choosing a therapist that isn't right for you in the first place, you maximize your chances of success.

You might have the name of two or three psychotherapists that seem like good possibilities. Perhaps the names have been given to you by a referral agency, a doctor, or a friend. Maybe you found the names on the Internet. Now you must choose between them. It can feel overwhelming to make that decision. You might feel vulnerable—even a bit intimidated. It is not unusual for someone to feel like he'd rather just pick up the phone and set up an appointment with the first name he comes across

Eric: Not Afraid to Ask Questions

Eric, a former patient of mine, explained how he almost picked the first person he came across, and why he changed his mind. Eric is a successful corporate tax attorney—not someone you would ordinarily think of as vulnerable or easily intimidated. He told me that interviewing prospective psychotherapists on the phone made him feel like a "presumptuous schoolkid." He felt he didn't really have the right to ask the therapist about his credentials and was worried that the therapist would be offended by his questions.

But because Eric's own tax clients often questioned him, even grilled him before setting up an appointment, he decided to follow their lead. He spent a total of three hours interviewing eight therapists. He told me that interviewing psychotherapists was one of "the smartest moves I ever made."

Eric is financially savvy. He saw therapy as a financial investment in his emotional future. "People spend more time deciding to buy a tie or deciding what restaurant to eat in. Don't let yourself fall into that trap," he advises. "Choose a therapist as carefully as you would a financial advisor or . . . a tax attorney!"

You have the right to ask a therapist questions. Don't be afraid that you will be setting up an adversarial relationship by doing so. If a therapist balks at answering any reasonable questions, you should regard his reluctance as a red flag. Thank the therapist for his or her time and seek help elsewhere. Remember, it will be far easier to do this now, over the phone, rather than later in person.

In fact, your questions can help the therapist too. An ethical therapist will respect your diligence in being proactive. It has been my experience that I gain additional respect for a patient that does his homework and asks tough questions. Hopefully, most professionals give the same high level of care to all patients, but it might be reasonable to assume that at least some therapists (subconsciously, perhaps) make an extra effort with patients who are informed and demand a higher standard of care from the outset.

The Initial Phone Interview

Some simple steps will help ensure that your phone interview accomplishes its goal. Some of these steps may seem obvious, but when you are feeling nervous or vulnerable, they can easily be forgotten, so be sure to review them before you begin each phone interview.

You will probably not be able to interview a therapist the first time you call. You will most likely have to schedule a phone interview in advance. When calling a therapist who works in a clinic, you may be able to schedule a phone appointment with him by speaking to a receptionist or secretary.

When calling a therapist in private practice, expect to leave him a voice mail message; he probably won't have a secretary or receptionist. Leave your name; just a first name is okay if you are uncomfortable sharing your full name. Don't worry—therapists are used to prospective patients wanting to remain anonymous. Don't forget, though, to leave a phone number and a good time for the therapist to call you back. Many therapists understand that you may be concerned about privacy and will not have their phone set to block private or anonymous calls if you prefer to dial a call that way.

When he does get back to you or if you do happen to reach him right away, tell him you have some questions about therapy and that you will need about ten minutes of his time. The phone interview should be between ten and twenty minutes long. Ask him when you can schedule a convenient time to speak.

During the phone interview, make sure you are sitting in a quiet place where you are not likely to be disturbed. If possible, use a landline rather than a cell phone—you'll probably have better reception. Have a pen handy. You may copy the phone interview sheet at the end of this chapter (Figure 3.1) and use it as a guide. At the start of the interview be sure to introduce yourself a bit more fully and tell the therapist how you heard about him. Let him know you are going to ask him a few questions that will help you decide whether or not to schedule an initial session with him.

Verifying Credentials

I recommend that the first topic of your phone interview should be about the therapist's credentials. When interviewing any therapist about his credentials, keep in mind that no one is an expert in treating every problem. Yes, there are some general principles and methods of psychotherapy that a professional can use in a broad variety of cases, but there will always be gaps in his knowledge and experience—there is just too much to learn that doesn't fall into the category of "general psychotherapy." Keep your eyes and ears open; if a psychotherapist says he is an expert in more than a couple of areas, investigate more fully. He may be someone with a very broad and deep range of clinical experience, or his experience might not be quite as all-encompassing as he says. *Clinical experience* is gleaned from working with patients in a clinical setting (as opposed to a classroom), such as a hospital or clinic, that is, treating patients either under supervision or on one's own.

In order to ensure that the psychotherapist you are thinking of hiring represents his clinical experience fairly, ask pointed questions and do your research before you schedule an appointment with him. You can start finding out about his experience by doing an Internet search—just type his name into your browser and see what comes up. Of course, he may only be listed on state registries, the details of which don't usually pop up on search engines. Also, not everything on the Internet is true, so try to rely on reputable sources like the websites of major organizations, such as the ones listed in the resources section at the back of this book, rather than blogs or chat rooms.

Even though you will most likely know (and hopefully research) what a psychotherapist's credentials are before you call him, it is important to *confirm this information during the phone interview*. Ask him which licenses and certifications he has and if they are up-to-date. Sometimes a therapist may not be up-to-date in his credentials and will not be legally able to treat patients. Alternately, he may have trained for and received a new credential in order to be able to treat a specific clinical issue. If you aren't sure what a credential means, ask the therapist for an explanation. If he gives you abbreviations or initials, ask what they stand for. Be sure to write down all terms so you can research them after the call if necessary.

Also, be sure to ask the therapist what sources you should contact in order to verify his credentials. He should give you a name and website or a phone number of a state agency or registry. Every state has a registry of professionals that keeps tracks of licenses and/or certifications. You can also contact the national professional associations listed in the resource guide at the end of this book and ask them how to contact your state's registry of professions. Don't just give this lip service. Follow through by calling, e-mailing, or logging on to the appropriate website to verify that the therapist's licenses and/or certifications are in order.

Alyssa: Uncovering Credential Fraud

A colleague of mine contacted me for advice about a case he had last year. A woman named Alyssa visited him in his office in a suburb of an East Coast city. She broke down in tears as she walked in the door. She had been going to family counseling along with her husband and two children. Her husband and teenage sons had drinking problems. She had been literally dragging them to therapy with a counselor who had been highly recommended by a member of a well-established religious organization she belonged to. Both she and her husband worked overtime in order to pay for the cost of the sessions since they weren't covered by their insurance.

The counselor had told them he was an addiction specialist and had the initials CASAC after his name. The credential was printed after his name on his business card, on his website, and in articles he had written for a newsletter they subscribed to. He also had recently published a book about adolescents and addiction, and had a list of approbations from a couple of people in the field, as well as leaders of Alyssa's community.

After six months of twice-weekly sessions, Alyssa saw no results. If anything, her husband's and sons' drinking became more frequent and more and more arguments erupted. One night, unable to sleep from worry, Alyssa logged on to the counselor's website and his blog corner. She thought that perhaps there were some blog posts that would be helpful. She didn't find anything new, so on a whim, she decided to find out more about what a CASAC credential actually entailed. She learned that most CASACs were connected with established substance abuse programs. She decided to find out if the counselor had worked with a treatment program in the past. By default, she finally logged on to the state substance abuse website, which was the name of the registry in her state, and began to search for the counselor's name on the CASAC list.

To her horror, Alyssa found out he was not a CASAC, and in fact had no verifiable certifications or licenses. The next day she called the registry. They said they were unable to tell her whether or not the counselor had ever been trained in the field at all. They recommended she give them the name of the counselor and his contact information, and also urged her to issue a formal complaint. Alyssa felt uncomfortable doing so since he had been recommended by several prominent members of her community. She also thought it might expose her family to embarrassment.

However, Alyssa really wanted to protect others who might see this man for "counseling." She felt comfortable enough (and angry enough) to ask him to remove the CASAC credentials from his website, which he promptly agreed to do because he feared exposure. She also asked for her money back, but he told her he didn't have "on hand" the nearly $6,000 she had paid him. Needless to say, Alyssa and her family didn't get back the time they lost, let alone the money. She finally wrote a letter to the organization that had made the recommendation and told them her story.

Perhaps the worst thing about this type of situation is that it can cause patients who could really benefit from psychotherapy to lose confidence in therapists and not seek help again. My guess is that the falsifying of credentials, though sensational, is probably rare. Alyssa's story does have a happy ending. The family actually drew closer together while trying to cope with this unfortunate incident. After the father and sons completed four months of a substance abuse treatment program, the family entered counseling together. Today, several months later, they are doing much better, though they will most likely continue therapy for two to three more months.

How Much Experience Should a Therapist Have?

It has been my experience that patients just don't ask enough questions about therapy and therapists before they come to therapy. You might feel a bit embarrassed asking questions about credentials, training, and experience, but I want to assure you that there are therapists who hope you will ask about our qualifications. We want patients to check us out before they hire us; this will help raise the standards for the profession as a whole.

One of the reasons you should ask a therapist about his credentials is that you want to be able to know he has had appropriate training and on-the-job experience. It is important that he is able to work with problems similar to those you face, whether it is anxiety, depression, anger, an addiction, an eating disorder, and so on. Of course, during the phone interview you will be giving the therapist your ideas and impressions about what is bothering you. You should also tell him about any previous diagnosis you may have had. After entering therapy, you may possibly end up addressing different problems than the one you originally contacted the therapist about, but the original information you give is still invaluable. Suffice it to say, in addition to any clinical description of your problem, it is important to give the therapist *your* best understanding of what is going on in your life.

For example, you might say, "I have a teenage son who is extremely rebellious and is not doing well in school. We are constantly arguing. Have you had any special training for this kind of problem?" Or, "I'm crying a lot and feeling that my life doesn't have much meaning; what training have you had that addresses these problems?"

When you articulate what you think the problem is, the therapist will be better able to tell you whether or not he has had the appropriate training. For example, if you think you have been experiencing panic attacks, ask the therapist specifically what kind of *training* (education, certifications, and/or internships) he has had that makes him able to treat panic attacks. In addition to special training, he should have attended a general university program or its equivalent. He should also have done an internship or other supervised training in a clinical setting like a hospital or outpatient clinic.

Ask him where he studied, what his degree is in, and when he graduated, and write down his answers. Later, you can verify this information by contacting the schools and programs he named. You might also want to verify some of this information by asking to see his diplomas, licenses, and certificates when you do end up scheduling an appointment with him. Don't worry: a qualified and competent therapist won't be offended in the least. He'll probably be delighted to dust off his licenses and certifications and take them down from the wall where they will most likely be hanging. Of course, he might be a bit surprised—after all, many patients are content with merely sneaking peeks at framed certificates and diplomas when they think we aren't looking.

Next, and more important, ask *how much* clinical experience a therapist has had treating people with issues similar to yours. For example, you can ask something like this: "How many years have you been treating defiant teenagers?" Or, "How many years have you been treating people with symptoms like mine?" He should be able to tell you the exact number of years he has been treating patients with similar problems. *A therapist should have at the very least one year's experience working extensively and directly with patients who have had problems similar to yours.* He should also be able to tell you the approximate number of patients he has treated who've faced similar issues. For example, you should feel comfortable asking him how many teenage patients he has treated with your son's problems, or how many patients with symptoms like yours.

I recommend that if you choose a therapist who has had only a year or two of general clinical experience, he should have successfully treated at least ten patients with problems similar to yours; more would be better. If, however, the therapist has had many years of clinical experience, but he's only treated five or so people with your specific problem, and treated them successfully, that might be good enough. His general experience, coupled with some expertise in addressing similar problems, will mean he can use his various clinical experiences to create viable treatment plans for diverse individual needs. Also, don't be surprised if a therapist can only give you an approximate number of patients he has treated with problems similar to yours (especially if the answer is in the hundreds or even thousands). Those of us with many years of experience generally don't know the exact number of patients we have worked with.

By asking the therapist to explain his ability to treat your particular problem before setting up an appointment, you will also be implying that you expect a certain standard of care. He will know you really want him to focus on your issues and not go off on tangents. He will be far less likely to just "move you along," and far more likely to really do the hard work necessary to help you get better.

Asking About Successful Outcomes

You will also want to ask the therapist about his *successful outcomes*. A therapist should be able to tell you what percentage (approximately) of his patients with problems similar to yours have achieved successful outcomes with his help. A successful outcome is the result of excellent treatment, the end result being patients who are able to leave therapy and live meaningful, productive, and positive lives without recurrence of serious symptoms or without having to return to therapy on a regular basis. A successful outcome may mean, for many patients, there is no need for therapy after the initial course of therapy; for those with mental illness, a successful outcome may mean learning how to manage symptoms but still attend limited and/or minimal therapy sessions.

Although his answer to the question about successful outcomes may be subjective and will rely heavily on his interpretation of events, you can learn a few things about the therapist if you read between the lines. His answer can tell you how diligent he is about following up with his patients. His answer can also give you clues about how he runs his practice.

Is he results-oriented, viewing successful outcomes as the main reason for therapy? Or is he process-oriented, focusing more on the value of the therapeutic process? Is he aware of the successes (or lack of success) he has had in his clinical work? Or is he not really in tune with his performance?

As a results-oriented therapist, I believe that, like any other service, *achieving a successful outcome is the main goal of therapy.* Therefore, I keep track of how my patients are doing, even after they have completed therapy. I follow up with a majority of my patients six months, one year, and even two years after they leave therapy. I keep careful records of positive responses as well as any negative ones. I especially try to follow up with patients who had very challenging problems, or problems with a high rate of relapse.

I am usually able to tell a prospective patient what percentage of my patients (including those with specific issues such as anxiety, depression, substance abuse problems, obsessive-compulsive disorder, post-traumatic stress syndrome, etc.) have had positive, long-lasting outcomes. Though this follow-up work is very time-consuming, I find it invaluable.

By following up, I am able to evaluate the methods I use and hone in on where I might need more training. I might find, for example, the need to consult with colleagues who have certain areas of expertise or research and read up on more of the latest information. All competent therapists continually seek feedback and opportunities to improve their skills.

Follow-up is also invaluable to my patients. They deserve to get the best care I can give. Like most therapists, I want to be able to help my patients reach their goals. Also, I really like being able to tell prospective patients what percentage of my cases show successful, long-lasting outcomes—because I am proud of that number!

If the therapist you are interviewing seems unwilling to answer your questions about training, experience, and outcomes, or says something like, "Well, every case is different," or "I can't give you answers until I meet you in person," then I suggest you tell him that you won't schedule an appointment unless you briefly discuss these topics. You might also want to let him know you are interviewing other therapists. *Don't be afraid to assert your right to know a therapist's qualifications before you give him a dime of your hard-earned money.*

If a therapist answers grudgingly or not at all or tries to intimidate you into meeting with him, remember—he will probably not be someone you will feel comfortable sharing your intimate thoughts with. Fortunately, those therapists who are qualified and competent will not be threatened by questions, and in fact will answer them graciously. Don't be intimidated by resistance and don't hesitate to get the facts. By not asking questions you run the risk, however small, of ending up with a therapist like Dorothy Jones.

Dorothy Jones: Playing with Letters

Dorothy Jones, as I will call her, is a social worker. Last year she graduated from a social work program. One day, not too long ago, a patient of mine named Martin brought in a weekly newspaper and showed me a full-color, glossy insert all about Dorothy Jones. Martin wanted to know if he should bring his eight-year-old daughter to her for testing, and asked my advice. I told him I would do a little research and get back to him.

The glossy insert contained a third-person announcement that Dorothy Jones was now a CEGP. (The initials and meaning used here have been altered but are similar in meaning to the original ones used by Ms. Jones.) It went on to say that after rigorous training, she was now a certified specialist and was entitled to be called a "children's emotional growth professional." This qualified her, according to the beautifully designed advertisement, to work with children and adolescents on any and all issues ranging from learning disabilities to eating disorders.

According to the insert, she was also now qualified to do a broad range of clinical testing, for which she charged $600 per hour, substantially above the rate most other professionals in her city charge for testing. "That's some impressive certification," I thought. It sounded like she did several years' worth of coursework; in fact, it sounded unusually grueling. I had never heard of a CEGP and neither had any of my colleagues—I asked around—so that night we researched it on the Internet.

What we found was surprising. There is no such certification as a CEGP. What we did find was a government agency with a subdivision with these initials. A CEGP was not, however, a training program or certification, just the name of a division of a government agency related to child care.

This began to smell really fishy. It seemed to us that any unsuspecting potential patient might type in the initials CEGP on their computer and come up with the link to an official government agency. It looked so impressive! Dorothy Jones was counting on them not to investigate any further. After some more digging around, we also found an online correspondence course called CEGP, which handed over a "certification" unapproved by any state or federal agency. The certification was for a course in play therapy specifically designed for children who were having problems bonding with peers or siblings. The website featured a disclaimer at the top that said the CEGP certificate awarded (after shelling out the $699 for completing an eight-hour Internet course) was not recognized by any state or national agency.

Dorothy had clearly taken the yellow brick road to an imaginary credential. She parlayed an eight-hour online course into a specialty in several childhood disorders. Because under her licensed master of social work (LMSW), she was legally allowed to work with kids with these disorders (as long as she got specialized training), she was doing nothing overtly illegal, no matter how unethical. Dorothy spent several thousand dollars advertising her newfound specialty and preyed upon parents when they were at their most vulnerable.

If Martin called Dorothy and asked about her education and training, and also verified the program she attended, he would have seen that she had essentially no more education or special training than any other LMSW fresh out of school, assuming she answered honestly. But we are willing to bet that if he had asked Dorothy about her outcomes, she would have hemmed and hawed and been unable to come up with a convincing figure.

When researching this book, we were told several stories similar to Martin's. The perpetrators were from a variety of professional therapy backgrounds, not just LMSWs. We chose to share this story with you because this kind of "soft" fraud could be easily carried out by any professional or nonprofessional. We don't want to suggest that LMSWs or any other type of psychotherapist is more prone to fraudulent behavior than another.

In general, most states require (or strongly suggest) that psychotherapists maintain continuing professional competence throughout their career. In many cases they must assess their professional abilities by self-evaluation and supervised peer consultation or tests. They should update and expand their knowledge and skills throughout their careers through continuing education and training programs (highly specialized credentials usually have specific continuing education requirements). Before using a modality not included in previous professional training, they must generally enroll in a course in a recognized institution and/or with recognized authorities on the subject and receive some type of certification that ensures competency.

The onus of following these ethical regulatory guidelines rests solely on the practitioner. Therefore, it is important to rely not only on what a therapist has to say about himself but also to find out what others have to say about him.

References and Reputation

Asking for references when hiring anyone to work for you (in any capacity) should be automatic. Actually checking the references out should also be automatic, but surprisingly, many people don't check references. They just don't believe that checking references is worth the effort. But we assure you it is.

When asking a therapist for references, listen to his response. He should quickly and pleasantly agree to give you some names of colleagues. In fact, he should be able to give you a name and title or two right away. Since many patients don't ask for references, therapists aren't used to supplying them. Therefore, they may not have their references' complete contact information handy, but they should be able to supply at least one name and get back to you within a day or two with the rest of the information.

It might feel strange to you to ask a therapist for a reference. You might not be comfortable with this, and you might be tempted to overlook this part of the interview. You may even be tempted to not check out the references that you are given. Many people feel better going with a therapist on a gut feeling, on faith. I respect gut feelings; they can be helpful, but they shouldn't replace doing the legwork.

What kind of reference should a therapist give you? Patients cannot be given as references. The federal codes governing confidentiality of therapy-patient interactions are catch-22's. They work in your favor—most of the time. It is comforting to know that your therapist cannot disclose information about you without a release signed by you. This process of releasing information to a third party is usually referred to as *informed consent;* that means that you have been informed of the exact nature, purpose, and extent of the disclosure, and that your permission can be rescinded at any time. This law is one of the best legal protections of your privacy that exists today.

When you are trying to find out information about a therapist, however, the confidentiality laws put you at a slight disadvantage. Because a therapist is unable to give you the name of any of his patients, this means that the therapist's "customers" can't tell you about his performance. (If a therapist offers patient references, not only is this highly irregular, it is illegal.) But there are other references he can give, and these can be even more meaningful than patient recommendations. These are references from other professionals. Psychotherapists work with a broad range of professionals, including medical doctors, educators, and other psychotherapists. I recommend that you ask for at least one professional reference. Remember, the therapist should be willing to supply you with references (graciously). If he balks at answering your request, cross his name off your list of potential therapists!

Any professional who has worked with the therapist is an appropriate reference. If the therapist has worked in a hospital or clinic setting, you may ask for the name of a supervisor or director, though some programs have policies that forbid the giving out of references. In addition to the name and title of the reference, be sure to ask his relationship to the therapist. Do they work together? Or do their kids have playdates occasionally? Ideally, the reference should be someone who can tell you about the therapist's professional life and clinical skills, not whether his kids prefer mac and cheese to pizza.

Usually, colleagues only give positive references. However, you can learn a lot by what remains unsaid. If a reference says, "Therapist A is a competent therapist, and he specializes in working with . . ." and no more, *but* he says that "Therapist B has achieved successful outcomes, and I send all my patients to him," you know that the reference has a high opinion of Therapist B and is not as enthusiastic about Therapist A. Of course, if the reference's kids are your therapist's kids' best friends, don't expect anything but praise. Even if that is the case, you can at least do some reading between the lines.

Also, a therapist's general reputation can be important, although it is not always a guarantee (as in the case of Alyssa and her family). You might want to call your primary care physician or other professional you know and ask them if they have heard of the therapist you are considering. Does he have a good reputation? Have they worked with him? Do they know anything about his outcomes or success rate? Remember, if they haven't heard of him, that doesn't mean he isn't good. An absence of information isn't evidence of poor skills.

Clinical Philosophy/Theoretical Orientation

After getting references, be sure to ask the therapist what his clinical style and/or clinical philosophy is. His answer should tell you how he generally likes to direct treatment. A *clinical philosophy* or *style* is the general approach a therapist subscribes to, believes in, and/or uses.

Give your therapist some time to think about this—he may be used to only answering this question when speaking with peers, and he might need a minute or two to "translate" his typical answer into "laypersonese."

There is no right or wrong answer. The answer just has to be something *you* are comfortable with. One therapist might say, "I find that confronting patients and really getting them to dig deep and examine their pasts is the best way to achieve success." Your personal response could be, "Wow. I like that gung-ho attitude." Or you might want to run for the hills.

Another therapist might say, "Generally I allow the patient to take the lead—I find a nonjudgmental approach works best." You might prefer this more gentle approach. One therapist might like to explore what the basis of your problem is right away. Another might like to address your feelings and behavior first and worry about the basis of the problem only down the road, if at all.

When answering your question, the therapist might use terms like *reality oriented* (therapy that focuses on counseling and problem solving in the here and now as well as offering instruction in how to create a better future); *behavioral oriented* (a treatment approach that aims to help patients substitute desirable behaviors for undesirable ones); *gestalt oriented* (a kind of therapy that focuses on the gaining of awareness of emotions and behaviors in the present rather than the past); or *patient centered* (any system of psychotherapy that assumes that the patient has the internal resources needed to improve and is the one who is in the best position to resolve his own problems). Ask the therapist to explain what these or any unfamiliar terms mean. Now's your chance to get a basic picture of this therapist's clinical viewpoints.

Don't be surprised if the therapist qualifies his statements by saying that he might change his style or technique depending on the issues that arise during therapy. This is quite common and a valid approach. Many therapists will say they like the patient to take the lead in certain areas and generally like to ask the patient what he would like to focus on and how much confrontation is comfortable for him.

By listening to a therapist's response, you will be better able to gauge if you will be comfortable with him or not. Being comfortable with a therapist leads to trusting a therapist, which then leads to developing the kind of relationship needed to help you achieve your therapeutic goals.

If you are comfortable with the therapist's answers so far, you can move on to the next topic. If not, you may want to ask the therapist to describe the specific techniques he uses. See if he mentions any of the accepted techniques described in Chapter 2. If he mentions a technique that you have never heard of, or whose efficacy you doubt, don't hesitate to contact a mental health professional association to find out if this is a recommended proven or evidence-based technique.

Ethics and Values

There is only one question early on that you need to ask in order to find out if a therapist has a high standard of ethics. And there is also only one correct answer. The question is: How will you know I am done with therapy? The correct answer will sound something like this: "We will know you are done with therapy when either we both feel that we have gone as far as we can go together and have achieved our goals, or when we reach a point in time (to be agreed upon in advance, such as a period of four to six months) where we both feel we aren't getting anywhere. If that is the case, we will talk about clinical alternatives, including treatment with a different therapist." Other answers, such as "When I determine you are better," "What—end therapy? I think you need to be in therapy for life!" or "When your insurance runs out" display a profound disregard for acceptable standards of ethics.

Related to ethics, and in fact overlapping them, is the topic of values. *Ethics* is conduct that is moral and principled, based on generally agreed-upon values. *Values* are the beliefs, conduct, and outlook regarded as positive by an individual, group, or culture. Suppose you have found a therapist with the credentials and training you need to help you. Suppose he has successfully treated hundreds of people with your problem over the course of a decade. Suppose his clinical style sounds warm and friendly to you—you can hardly wait to open up and tell him what's bothering you. You feel he could really help. And then suppose you mention your value system.

Maybe you tell him that you are an Evangelical Christian, or an atheist, a liberal, a conservative, a hunter, or a vegetarian. Or that you subscribe to any other belief system or way of life that may not be too common in your neck of the woods. Does the therapist effectively say, "So what?" That is a great answer. Or does he say, "I have worked with many people who are fruitarians; this is not a problem at all."? Even better. Or does he become silent, sound repulsed, or tell you he can "treat you for that problem"?

If he views your genuine values or belief system as wrong or something that needs to be corrected, he won't be the right therapist for you. Of course, in some instances you may want to address certain behaviors you are participating in that actually conflict with your values—that is something certainly worth mentioning to a therapist during the phone interview or during your first session or two, if possible.

In order to avoid conflict down the road, I recommend you tell a therapist over the phone about your sexuality, religious beliefs, or any disabilities you may have if you believe they could be considered controversial or make some people feel uncomfortable. Still, the therapist should not sound shocked or disapproving. He should be able to respond by saying he works with and respects all types of patients or he should refer you to someone you would be more comfortable with. A lack of respect for your value system could be a most unwelcome deal breaker down the road.

Balance of Professionalism and Personality

Although ideally you will find a therapist with excellent credentials, appropriate training, and relevant experience, as well as a very high percentage of successful outcomes, therapy will simply not succeed if you dislike the therapist or don't trust him. Therefore, you must find a therapist who has a good balance of professional attributes and personality. Concerning personality, you should put at least some trust in your gut feelings. If you would like a more concrete way to assess personality, the following information may help.

During the phone interview, pay attention to how the therapist interacts with you. If he cuts you off when you are speaking or forcefully tells you what to do, chances are he won't be someone you can work with. Is he courteous? Is he friendly but professional? Does he listen to you and respond to your questions and concerns? You should be able to answer, "Yes."

You might be better able to evaluate whether or not this therapist's personality is a good match for you if you "keep score." Take the time to fill in the personality section of the phone interview checklist immediately after the phone call. Be sure to factor in whether or not you liked, disliked, or felt neutral about each therapist you interview.

Fees and Hours

Although I suggest you complete the parts of the phone interview in the order listed, you can be more flexible when it comes to asking about fees. You may ask a therapist about his fees at the beginning or end of the phone interview or somewhere in between. He might mention his fees right up front. By the time you hang up the phone, be sure you understand what his fees are per one-hour session. Some therapists have fifty-minute session times so they can write notes during the remaining ten minutes. I dislike this practice because I feel that ten minutes is your time, and is usually necessary.

Ask how lenient he will be about charging more if a session runs over the allotted time. Will he charge you for missed sessions? How much notice does he need if you need to cancel a session? What about emergencies? Also ask how much he will charge if you have to talk to him on the phone. Usually if you just need a couple of minutes to check in with your therapist, he won't charge you. Remember, if you or a family member need to talk for more than a couple of minutes, unless it is a life-threatening emergency, it is only reasonable for you to schedule an office appointment (or a phone appointment if there is absolutely no alternative) and pay for the therapist's time.

If his fee is impossible to fit into your budget, ask if he has a sliding scale—but be fair. A colleague of mine discounted her fees substantially in order to do marriage and family counseling with a family that was referred to her by a hospital in which she worked. She was disappointed to learn from the teenage kids that the family owned two homes, skied in the Austrian Alps each winter, and had a live-in maid. When she asked the parents if this was true, they said yes, but that they just couldn't find the money for therapy in their budget. Since then, my colleague only offers a reduced fee if she sees a tax return, two pay stubs, and a copy of the family budget. Remember, if you want to benefit from a sliding-scale rate, don't take it personally if your therapist asks for a confirmation of your income.

A therapist should be excited about working with a new patient. Sometimes, waiting to discuss fees until the end of the phone interview can be to your advantage, especially if the therapist is excited about working with you after learning a bit about you. If he believes strongly that he can help you, he might be willing to accept a lower fee if you are in a tough financial position. Be prepared, though, to show pay stubs and/or your tax return.

Also, if you have time restrictions (you are only free nights or weekends, for example), you should let the therapist know right away. Most therapists do have at least some weekend and evening hours. Many even have those hours exclusively set aside for their private practices because they work at a hospital or clinic during the day. Make sure the therapist has hours that are compatible with your schedule.

Decisions, Decisions, Decisions

Unless you are truly 100 percent sure this is the right therapist for you and definitely want to schedule an appointment, I recommend that at the conclusion of the phone interview you thank the therapist for his time without scheduling a session. Tell him you will be deciding within a few days whether or not you want to set up an initial appointment with him.

Be sure to make any special notes to yourself about the therapist on the interview sheet right after you hang up the phone. Otherwise, you are likely to forget what you were thinking and feeling. If the therapist impressed you in an area, go ahead and give him a star, smiley face, or an A. If you had any concerns, draw in a red flag or a question mark. Jot down any questions you may have. Also, check references right away while the conversation is still fresh in your mind. If rating your overall impression of the therapist on a scale of 1–10 is helpful to you, go ahead and do so.

Now, the hard part begins. It is possible that if you have interviewed two or three therapists, you already have an idea who the best candidate would be. But if you have interviewed more than three, you may have a harder time deciding. Read the interview sheets again. Compare them side by side. Is one candidate a superstar when it comes to experience, but his clinical style left you cold? Do you really like a candidate's personality but aren't so pleased that he is fresh out of school and sounds inexperienced? Evaluating which therapist you should see may be difficult, but it's not, as they say, rocket science. Try to make sure that the therapist you choose has an acceptable level of each of the qualities you seek, but don't expect him to fully maximize every quality you would like to find.

When you've decided which therapist to schedule a session with, call and set up your first appointment—and don't forget to ask for directions to his office! Remember, setting up a therapy session is not a contractual obligation. If after one or more sessions, the therapist displays unprofessional behavior or you are extremely uncomfortable with your choice, you are free to choose to work with someone else. But keep in mind that psychotherapy can be an uncomfortable or difficult experience. Throughout this book, we will help you differentiate between therapy that feels uncomfortable because it is working and therapy that feels uncomfortable because it is bad therapy.

Figure 3.1. Phone Interview Checklist

Date: _____ Time of Interview: _____
Name of Therapist: _____

1. Credentials
- Credential _____ Verification _____
- Credential _____ Verification _____
- Credential _____ Verification _____

2. Training, Clinical Experience, and Outcomes
- Education _____
  _____
  _____
- Training _____
  _____
  _____
- Experience with your specific issue _____
  _____
  _____
  - Number of years experience treating specific issue _____
  - Number of patients treated with specific issue (approximately) _____
- Percentage of Successful Outcomes _____

3. References and Reputation
  A. _____
  B. _____
  C. _____
  Notes: _____
  _____

4. Clinical Philosophy
  _____
  _____

_____

_____

Terms Used: _____

_____

_____

5. Ethics Question

How will I know when therapy is completed?

Therapist's Answer: _____

_____

_____

_____

6. My Values and Belief (I am, I believe, etc.): _____

_____

_____

_____

Therapist's feedback about my values and beliefs: _____

_____

_____

_____

Accepting of my values and beliefs: ❑ Yes ❑ No

7. Personality

- Therapist let me complete sentences and was polite.   ❑ Yes ❑ No
- Therapist gave me agreed-upon allotted time for call.   ❑ Yes ❑ No
- Therapist had the right amount of forcefulness and   ❑ Yes ❑ No
  gentleness for me.
- I liked talking and listening to him over the phone.   ❑ Yes ❑ No

8. Fees and Hours

Fees:

- There is/is not a sliding scale   ❑ Yes ❑ No
- Each session lasts _____ hours and costs $_____

- The initial evaluation fee is $_____
- I can afford the fee per session (assume you will see the   ❏ Yes ❏ No
  therapist once a week or every other week)
- There is a fee if a session runs over   ❏ Yes ❏ No
- There is a fee for occasional phone calls   ❏ Yes ❏ No
- The therapist needs _____ hours'/days' notice to
  cancel/reschedule missed sessions   ❏ Yes ❏ No
- There is a charge for missed sessions   ❏ Yes ❏ No

Hours:

- The therapist has hours that are compatible with mine   ❏ Yes ❏ No
- Office Hours are:

Sunday: _____ Monday: _____ Tuesday: _____ Wednesday: _____

Thursday: _____ Friday: _____ Saturday: _____

Notes: _____

_____

_____

_____

_____

_____

Chapter 4

FOCUS ON YOUR FIRST APPOINTMENT

If you understand the beginning well, the end will not trouble you.

—PROVERB FROM THE ASHANTI PEOPLE OF GHANA

It goes without saying that you should get directions to the therapist's office and also allow plenty of travel time for your first appointment. Why? Because when you are stressed or nervous, it's hard to think of the practical, little stuff until you are hit with it—and you find yourself frantically looking for a parking spot or getting on the wrong bus. Remember, if you forgot to ask the therapist for directions during the phone interview, use a map, mapquest.com, a GPS, or your local public transportation's website. If you're late, you may not get your full hour-long session as your therapist will most likely end your session at the appointed time—otherwise he will be late for his next patient.

Like most people, you've probably spent way too much time waiting in doctors' or dentists' offices, but you probably won't have to wait long to see your therapist. Because psychotherapists treat fewer patients per day than doctors do, generally don't overbook appointments, and also block off an entire hour to see each patient, they usually run on time.

Like you, the therapist should try to be punctual. However, sometimes patient emergencies could cause him to run late. If that's the case, he should step into the waiting room and ask if you mind waiting a specified amount of time—he shouldn't just assume you'll wait. Your time is valuable, too. If the wait seems excessive and you do mind waiting longer, tell him you would rather reschedule.

A therapist's overall punctuality (throughout the course of therapy) is indicative of how much he respects his patients and values their feelings. So many patients we interviewed (like Madeline in Chapter 7) told us stories about the chronic lateness of their therapists that we could have written a chapter about this subject alone. Sometimes people who are chronically late are late because forcing people to wait is a way to control them emotionally. It makes many people feel upset and vulnerable to be kept waiting. Of course, there are many different reasons anyone, including your psychotherapist, can run late. And yes, occasionally, everyone runs late, but we don't believe that it should happen with any regularity.

First Impressions: What to Look For

On the rare occasion when your therapist is running late, you might find it helpful if the waiting room is as comfortable and relaxing as possible. There might be magazines or books for you to read, and the room should be reasonably clean. Clinics often have large waiting rooms, but therapists in private practice most likely will have small ones. Many therapists hang pictures on the walls, decorate with rugs and upholstery in soothing colors and soft textures, and arrange potted plants, an aquarium, or even a television in the waiting room. The ambiance of the waiting room should be relatively pleasant; the office where therapy takes place, more so. However, if your therapist doesn't have an aesthetic flair, don't let it distract you from the main purpose of a waiting room—a place to wait before you begin your session.

Whenever possible, a waiting room should be designed to protect your privacy. When being treated by a therapist in private practice you can reasonably expect to be able to arrive five to ten minutes before your appointment time and find the waiting room empty and the next patient either already gone or able to leave through a separate exit. Though therapists usually try to rent offices with two entrances, this may not always be possible. If no separate exit is available, therapists should make every effort (barring emergencies) to schedule appointments with at least ten- to fifteen-minute breaks in between patients. They should be using that break time to write detailed notes about the previous patient's session, something you will learn more about later in this chapter.

If you are very concerned about privacy, or your therapist doesn't have the facilities or the schedule that will allow you to remain as anonymous as you'd like, you could look for a therapist out of town, something some patients prefer to do. And if anonymity is a pressing concern for you, I suggest you avoid clinics where patients often sit in one large waiting room, and everyone can see everyone else.

Finally, the moment has arrived. The therapist shows you into his office. Some therapists like to shake hands; others greet patients with a warm hello. If you are uncomfortable shaking hands, let your therapist know right away. Don't worry—therapists are used to people expressing their inner thoughts and feelings and won't be offended by this. After greeting you, the therapist should offer you a comfortable chair or sofa to sit on.

The office, like the waiting room, should be clean. There will most likely be a desk, but the therapist, depending on his clinical style, may or may not sit behind it during a therapy session. Or he may begin working with a new patient from behind his desk then later ask if it would be okay if he moved to another spot in the room. Wherever he sits, it should be a comfortable distance away from you, and generally speaking, not within touching distance, at least not during the first appointment.

Some therapists never touch patients at all, while others occasionally pat a patient's hand or shoulder or shake hands. I believe that hugs are always inappropriate, especially with patients of the opposite sex, though a few therapists disagree. Whatever kinds of encouraging, respectful touch might occur, the therapist should ask your permission first. Needless to say, all touch must be nonsexual. Because touch can be misinterpreted and also because establishing healthy personal boundaries is often a goal of therapy, many therapists, including me, make a practice of limiting touch to the very occasional shaking of hands.

The therapist should be dressed in a way that isn't distracting to you, and in a way that gives you confidence in his professionalism. His hygiene should be good—you shouldn't think twice about his cleanliness. There should be no controversial slogans, political or otherwise, on a therapist's clothing (or on his walls, for that matter). He should be dressed as appropriately as any other professional in your town.

Obviously, a therapist in Papeete, Tahiti, might dress somewhat differently than one in Anchorage, Alaska, but my opinion is that a therapist's clothes should always be somewhat conservative and professional. Visible tattoos, piercings, or torn or dirty clothing are not, at least to me, confidence-inspiring. Your favorite musician might have a flamboyant appearance, but if your heart surgeon dressed like a pop star, would you think twice about going under the knife? I know I would. I believe you should apply those same standards to a therapist. A therapist who is trying to attract attention by making a shocking or overtly trendy statement with his or her dress is a therapist who is very possibly not mature enough to help you.

If you are the type of person who finds conservative or professional dress off-putting and would feel more relaxed if your therapist wore jeans and T-shirts, by all means, seek a therapist who makes *you* feel comfortable. You can let your feelings be your guide in this area, though I would encourage you to work with a therapist for at least a few sessions if your only complaint is that you found his conservative attire bothersome. You might find that after an appointment or two, his suit becomes "invisible."

The one absolute rule about clothing I would encourage you to adhere to is to *never* work with a therapist whose clothing is overtly seductive or immodest. An appearance designed to entice or seduce could very well mean that your therapist has issues with appropriate boundaries. Also, he or she could possibly be trying to manipulate or control others, including you. Any therapist, male or female, should dress modestly. Tight, revealing, or low-cut tops, very short skirts, high heels, tight pants, short shorts, heavy makeup, very heavy perfume or cologne, and so on are all good indications that your therapist is interested in attracting inappropriate attention. Obviously, enticing or seducing patients is strictly forbidden for any therapy professional, but unfortunately there have been rare cases where this has occurred.

As we mentioned, patients are in a vulnerable position, especially when they first come to therapy, and feelings of physical attraction can be distracting, confusing, and even overwhelming. These feelings are also easily confused with feelings of love. Physical attraction may lead a patient to be either more or less open and honest with the therapist than is beneficial. If your therapist is overtly seductive, you might consciously or subconsciously try to impress him by not revealing issues important to your clinical success. Or you might focus on some intimate details of your life while neglecting other important issues.

A Closer Look at Licenses

If you are comfortable, go ahead and take a look at the therapist's credentials (you should have begun this process already by checking with various regulating agencies after your phone interview). After the therapist greets you and shows you into his office, take a moment and ask to see his licenses and/or certifications. Remember, therapy patients who haven't read this book probably know far more about their lawyer's or dermatologist's qualifications than their therapist's. Yet a therapist is the person they are willing to trust with their most intimate thoughts and feelings! Many people find it easier to confide intimate secrets to others than share their bank balances. You should value your private thoughts and feelings at least as much as your bank balance, and you should share them only with those who are trustworthy.

Don't let shyness or fear get in your way—advocate for yourself right from the very first meeting. "Would you mind if I took a few moments to look at your credentials?" would be a good way to begin. The therapist should agree immediately and allow you to examine them. A therapist with a healthy ego and a good dose of humility won't in the least mind being questioned about his qualifications.

Most therapists display their credentials in the form of framed degrees, licenses, and certificates on a wall either behind their desks or elsewhere in the office. Make sure the degrees, licenses, and certificates are the same as what you were told over the phone. Also, in the case of certificates and licenses, make sure they're up-to-date. Some credentials may require periodic retesting, ongoing coursework, or the payment of renewal fees. Make sure the licenses or certificates are valid in the state in which the therapist is practicing—your therapist might be licensed to practice marriage and family counseling in North Dakota but not in North Carolina, where you live. If there is a discrepancy, this could indicate a problem. Also, if you are seeing a therapist for a special issue, such as an eating disorder or addiction, make sure he has a credential or training that supports treatment in that area. If at any point you are unsure of what any of his licenses or certificates really represent, or if they are relevant to your problem, go ahead and ask him to explain them.

If the therapist mentions that he has special training in an area, whether he tells you so on the phone, publishes it in an advertisement, or prints it on a business card, rest assured that it is appropriate for you to ask to see the relevant credential. You can phrase the request something like this: "You mentioned to me that you have special training in _____ (addiction, eating disorders, phobias, etc.). May I see the certificate or license that shows where and when you received this training?" Again, an ethical therapist won't balk—he will show you the credential if it is on hand (he may have it in a desk drawer, at another office, or elsewhere; if he does, he should offer to bring it in the next time you meet, and do so). Of course, he will have received some specialized training "on the job," so it's possible that he won't have a license or certificate for every area of specialization.

If you visually inspect a college or university degree, it is important to note that the therapist's B.A., M.A., or Ph.D. is in the field in which he is practicing. On occasion, a licensed counselor might get a Ph.D. in another area, such as biology, history, or a foreign language. He might already have an acceptable nondoctoral degree in counseling or social work and is therefore entitled to do psychotherapy. But it is unethical (though not overtly illegal) if he *implies* that his doctorate is in an area related to psychotherapy if it's an unrelated field, such as religious studies or physical therapy. If he expects you to call him "Dr.," or if there is a Ph.D. after his name, check and see where and in what field of study he earned his Ph.D. (In fact, it is important to check that a B.A. or M.A. are in an appropriate field as well.)

Recently it was brought to my attention by a member of a professional association that some counselors are getting easy and inexpensive online doctoral degrees in theology. They are doing this, according to my colleague, so they can put the letters Ph.D. after their names in order to charge more per session and create the illusion that they are able to treat a broader range of problems than they really are qualified to do. Could a therapist who uses an advanced degree in this manner still be a good counselor? Conceivably, he could, but anyone who is willing to misrepresent himself, however slightly, in order to charge more money and get more patients is, in my opinion, someone who is not really trustworthy. Integrity is important in any field; in psychotherapy it is imperative.

If, as you are looking at the credentials, you find names of schools you have never heard of, such as Shorty's School of Plumbing and Psychiatry, or licenses you are unfamiliar with, such as a license to practice Aqua Pilates Social Work, go ahead and write down the unfamiliar name. After the session you can do some more research online or make some phone calls to agencies or associations. That way, you won't end up like Simone.

Simone: Checking Qualifications

Simone is a teacher of English as a second language (ESL) whom the court system mandated to come for substance abuse treatment—she had been caught driving while under the influence of painkillers. She informed me that she was already in treatment with several specialists: a physical therapist for pain from a work injury, a doctor who originally prescribed the pain medication to which she had become addicted, and a psychotherapist who had been treating her for anxiety and depression for a period of four months.

I asked Simone to sign a release so we could discuss her case with her psychotherapist. Talia, the addiction counselor who I assigned to Simone's case, told me that when she looked up the phone number of the psychotherapist in a phone book, he was listed as a "hypnotherapist"—not recognized as a separate licensed psychotherapeutic profession in New York State. Hypnotherapy (the therapeutic use of hypnosis) can be a useful technique in certain kinds of therapy. Each state has different laws governing the various techniques used in therapy, as well as different laws governing which professions are recognized as types of psychotherapy and which aren't. I was hopeful that he had other credentials, and that hypnotherapy was used merely as an adjunct to his other clinical skills, in which case it could certainly be effective.

Talia suggested to Simone that the next time she visited her psychotherapist, she write down the name of the school or schools the therapist attended, as well as any licenses or certificates he might have. Talia told Simone that if our program was going to work with her,

we had to have full knowledge of her therapist's professional creden-
tials. The following week Simone returned. She handed over a piece of
paper upon which was written "Emblem International School of Hyp-
nosis" (we changed the name of the school here).

Simone reported that when she asked her therapist for the name of
the school he went to, he sheepishly pointed to a "degree" hanging on the
wall of his office. It was mounted in a very grand, very large, gilt
frame. But it was the only "credential" he offered to show her. She was
pretty upset when she learned he didn't have a license, degree, or equiv-
alent experience at all, and this online computer course in hypnosis
was the only "training" he'd had.

I am sorry to say that my clinic's encounter with Simone's "therapist" wasn't the only encounter we've had like this—through the years we have seen similar situations, which is why I emphatically encourage you to actively research your therapist's qualifications before you even meet. A therapist should be transparent about his professional credentials and there should never be a sense of mystery about what those credentials are.

In short, you are looking to make sure the therapist is who he says he is. You are looking to make sure his degrees, licenses, or certifications are from reputable schools, training programs, or agencies. You want to confirm that his credentials are appropriate and related to his area of specialty. You want to make sure he did not get the bulk of his education over the Internet (which may be fine for accounting or computer studies, but is *not* appropri- ate for a field where interaction with people is paramount—though some professionals disagree with me about this), or worse, get his degree (B.A., M.A., or Ph.D.) from a school that doesn't exist except in cyberspace. If an online school has an ".edu" at the end of the web address, if there is a school requirement to take core curriculum courses on campus, and if students have access to credentialed instructors whenever they have questions, then the education, and therefore the degree, might have some merit.

Bear in mind that many types of continuing education courses that professionals take to further their education—rather than learn the fundamentals—are often available online. Committed therapists often choose to continue to learn more about their field throughout their careers, and online classes can add to their skills and knowledge base, which is actually a plus.

Of course, most psychotherapists have their credentials in order. And most will be happy to let you see them. In fact, asking to see the actual printed credentials—again, preferably mentioning this in advance during the phone interview—can be an icebreaker during your first visit. Talking about a subject other than yourself can give you time to get to know the therapist and become acclimated to his office.

Getting to Know You

The first thing the therapist will most likely ask you is "What led you to come see me?" If you aren't sure where to begin or how to answer, I suggest you phrase your answer like this: "I have been having problems with _____ and I want to find out if therapy is the right course of action for me to take, and if you are the right therapist for me to work with." That way, you let the therapist know right away that you are viewing this first session not only as a therapy session but also as an exploratory session that will help you decide if he is the right therapist for you.

You don't have to feel an overwhelming connection with your therapist when you first meet, but you should get a sense that he is warm, caring, considerate, kind, encouraging, empathetic, and respectful. Yes, all those attributes sound like a tall order, but, frankly, anyone who enters the field of psychotherapy should possess (or work hard to develop), all of them.

During the first few appointments the therapist should ask a lot of questions and do a lot of listening. I can't stress enough how important it is that the therapist initially ask a lot of questions about you and your life. I would be very wary of a therapist who doesn't flood you with questions (and, of course, listen carefully to your answers without interrupting you). The therapist needs to understand who you are and why you are in therapy.

By asking focused questions, the therapist will be able to clear obstructions from your therapeutic path and help you chart a direct route to wellness. By listening carefully to your answers, maintaining eye contact, and appearing (and being) interested in you, the therapist will also be demonstrating that he understands the depth and the breadth of your answers. In the first few sessions, he should work hard to get a real understanding of who you are and what you want to accomplish in therapy.

Some therapists do not use this approach. Some therapists, especially those who practice psychoanalysis and its variants, believe that the patient should generate all information and figure out all the solutions to his problems himself. They allow the patient to talk about whatever he wishes. Then at the end of the session, psychoanalysts offer psychological explanations for what the patient just told them, or offer a few ideas or comments. Although I believe that it can work with the right patient, I feel this approach has limited use. I wouldn't go as far as the embittered Austrian satirist Karl Kraus, who said, "Psychoanalysis is that mental illness for which it regards itself a therapy." However, psychoanalysis and most of its offshoots are not able to offer empirical evidence that they help effect a positive outcome.

Patient-centered therapy (see Chapter 3), which includes techniques where the therapist asks questions, empathizes, and clarifies what a patient has just said in order to propel the patient forward to solve his own problems, does have plenty of empirical evidence that it is effective. In patient-centered therapy the practitioner may ask, "What do *you* think about what you just said?" The success of this type of therapy has been replicated in scientifically conducted experiments and well documented. I believe that this kind of interaction is also comfortable for most patients.

A therapist should not only make every effort to be involved with and help his patient, the patient should be able to clearly perceive this. The strict use of psychoanalytic techniques can cause you to question if the therapist is actually working to help you. As a patient, your perceptions are extremely important and can influence the outcome of therapy. Obviously, therapists who aren't perceived by their patients as caring and interested will most likely not make significant treatment gains. Of course, by asking questions about a therapist's clinical philosophy over the phone, you will already know whether or not the therapist uses a form of therapy that you feel comfortable trying.

Another thing to be aware of is what the therapist says or doesn't say during those times when he is *not* asking questions. He should generally not disclose personal information about himself except in certain specific instances where it may have therapeutic value. He should also never speak about another patient, *even if he doesn't mention the patient's name.* He may say, in a global way, "I have treated patients with issues similar to yours," but otherwise he should not speak about his cases. There are a few reasons that these kinds of behavior are unprofessional. In the story of Nick and Jessica, told to me by a couple seeking a referral for counseling, the problems with this are clearly illustrated.

Nick and Jessica: Disclosing Personal Information About Other Patients

Nick and Jessica Franklin, a recently married couple in their thirties, moved to a small college town four months after they got married, and between the pressure of the move and financial stress—Nick's accounting firm downsized shortly after they moved, and Jessica was just starting up a practice as a chiropractor—they began having arguments. They decided to go to a well-known marriage and family therapist who advertised heavily and cohosted a call-in show on a local radio station with her psychotherapist husband.

Throughout the sessions the therapist not only spoke about herself frequently, but once Nick and Jessica told her about their difficulties, she appeared to almost immediately lose interest in their problems. She began to share intimate details about her other patients' marital difficulties. Though she didn't say the names of the other patients, she gave enough identifying details that if the couple hadn't been new to the town, they would have likely been able to guess who the other patients were. She even discussed one of her husband's patients with them, mentioning what the person did for a living. Of course, this didn't exactly inspire their confidence in the therapist's ability to keep their sessions confidential. After a couple of sessions, they began to see that they weren't being helped at all—essentially they were paying the therapist to work out her own issues and gossip about her other patients. As soon as they realized this, they discontinued therapy and called me to ask for a referral to someone else.

Me, Myself, and I

Personality is important, as I have already mentioned. Your therapist should have a personality that you find pleasant to be around—at least for the duration of each session. However, in Western culture, and especially in the United States, we have various cults of personality, such as those related to celebrities or politicians. We are used to the media helping to create larger-than-life public figures, and have grown somewhat comfortable with arrogance parading as all-knowing beneficence and charm. It is important that a therapist be appealing to you in a general way, of course, but if a therapist is overwhelmingly charismatic and talks about you and your life in terms of himself, or tells you that you need to have no one else in your life but him, or promises to be your "savior," find another therapist—fast.

Sometimes people with a desire for power over others enter the field of psychotherapy. It isn't unheard of. Since many educational programs in the field require that students undergo some form of psychotherapy themselves, many people with inappropriate motives or confounding issues don't want to be exposed and decide to drop out of the field. However, occasionally those who are very good at manipulating others or presenting a false front can, and do, receive their degrees and licenses. Don't let this remote possibility deter you. I am a worse-case-scenario kind of thinker. I believe it is better to be educated and prepared for any eventuality. If you know what can go wrong, you can learn what to avoid. That being said, the majority of psychotherapists are motivated by a genuine desire to help others. They really care.

Empathy

Good therapists often have tremendous empathy for their patients in part because as part of their training, virtually all of them have gone through therapy, or at least an in-depth therapeutic evaluation, themselves. If you feel it is important to you to know more, you could ask the therapist if he has ever been in therapy himself, and, if so, when. You can phrase it like this: "Have you ever been in the therapeutic process yourself? And may I ask you how it worked out? What was your experience?" He will most likely answer that he went through therapy during his education, and that answer is to be expected. If he says he is currently in therapy, or has been in therapy very recently, I would question whether or not the therapist is ready to treat patients. He may be working out his own issues during your therapy sessions—to your detriment. Like anyone else, some therapists who have unresolved issues carry them into other areas of their lives, including their clinical practice. A therapist must have the closets of his psyche cleaned out and in order; of course, there may be a psychological dust ball here or there (no one is perfect) but overall, order and clarity should be the rule.

If you broke a thumb and you went to a medical doctor who also had a broken thumb, he could still diagnose you and most likely even treat you (unless, of course, you needed surgery!). But if you were dealing with issues of a broken marriage and your therapist, too, was dealing with issues of his broken marriage that could present a big problem. His personal issues could cloud his effectiveness, as he would be continually reminded of his own marital problems as he listened to you. Your therapy sessions may be the vehicle through which he is able to untangle his issues, but that is not what your therapy should be about—it should be about you, not the therapist.

The Biopsychosocial History/Evaluation

Not too far into your first session, usually right after you tell the therapist why you came to see him, the therapist will begin to do an *evaluation*— an initial and/or ongoing assessment of a patient's clinical status that will be used to develop a plan for treatment. The evaluation primarily includes a large body of information called the *biopsychosocial history*. This evaluation will help him gather specific information about you, including biographical, psychological, and social information (in far more detail than just general questions) and will help him understand you better. It will help him develop a detailed treatment plan based on your individual needs.

The therapist should write down your answers to the evaluation questions. Virtually any therapist who does not do a comprehensive written evaluation—unless you have given him permission to tape-record the information instead—or take detailed notes during sessions will be unable to remember important details about you. A psychotherapist is required to keep written treatment records of each patient. This is not only to facilitate treatment, but also for insurance reasons, in case he is asked by you to turn the case over to another doctor for medical reasons, or in case you want copies of your own records, which you are entitled to by law. If your therapist is not writing notes during (and after) your session, the chances are his treatment records will be sparse. Also, he will be unable to go over those all-important notes in order to refresh his memory before his next session with you. This will make treatment decisions very difficult.

Biographical Data

The first set of questions in the evaluation will include basic biographical data about you: your name, age, address, phone, birthday, education level, family information, emergency contact information, employment, and so on.

Substance Abuse History/Mental Health History

The next set of questions will either establish your history of alcohol/drug use or your mental health history. My preference (and my bias) is to do an alcohol and drug history first; if substance abuse or active addiction issues are present, they will be the first things that need to be addressed, as the presence of unresolved substance abuse or addiction will prevent psychotherapy from being effective.

Substance abuse is the harmful use of substances, including legal and illegal drugs, alcohol, and/or chemicals such as solvents or glue in order to alter a person's mood. Abuse of a prescribed or otherwise legal medication can occur when a patient uses more of the substance at a greater frequency than is required or prescribed. Additionally, abuse can occur when a person begins to build up tolerance to a medication or alcohol. Substance abuse of legal and illegal drugs, chemicals, alcohol, and even food and gambling can lead to dependency, also known as addiction.

Addiction (or *dependency*) is a psychological and physical disease in which a person has a dependency on legal or illegal drugs or alcohol, chemical solvents, harmful behaviors such as binging and purging on food, gambling, promiscuous sex, or other risky, dangerous behaviors. When an individual is dependent on a dangerous chemical or behavior, he feels compelled to indulge in the drug or behavior to relieve uncomfortable feelings and symptoms, such as anxiety or nervousness, while disregarding the dangerous consequences. Addiction may drive a person to lie, cheat, and steal to cover up his addiction or to get the resources to indulge in his addiction. It is one of the most devastating of diseases and affects the individual and his family, coworkers, community, and society at large. Though there are some schools of thought that addiction is strictly a moral problem and not a disease, those models do not offer any empirically effective treatment, while the disease model does offer various modes of successful treatment.

The bottom line is that a lot of mental health issues can be attributed to the use of illegal or even legal substances, such as prescription drugs or liquor. If the therapist can establish before he even gets to the mental health questions that chemicals are causing or exacerbating symptoms of emotional or mental illness, then he can zoom right in on the problem.

The therapist should have a list of specific frequently abused substances from your state or from the federal Substance Abuse and Mental Health Services Administration (SAMHSA), an excellent resource listed in the back of this book. In fact, SAMHSA, which is one of the more effective federal programs, acknowledges by its very name that substance abuse has primacy in the national discussion about mental health.

My belief, actually my wish, is that all psychologists and social workers would always ask questions about substance abuse. They really need to do so at the beginning of treatment. Currently, many don't, unless they have special addiction training, which has fostered awareness of this problem.

SAMHSA estimates that at least 7 to 10 million Americans have a serious mental illness in some way related to chemical substance usage—either they are using drugs or alcohol to help *alleviate* their psychological symptoms, or the drugs or alcohol are *causing* their symptoms. The figures for those who have less serious emotional problems—like *minor* depression or anxiety—and who are also substance abusers vary widely, but an educated guess would be that it is at least ten times the amount of those with *serious* mental illness that is chemically related. So many patients regularly medicate themselves with culturally acceptable substances from cabernet to cough syrup that it is vitally important that all therapists learn to take a drug and alcohol history from their patients. Every therapist should also cultivate relationships with some good addiction programs to which he can refer patients. Otherwise, patients like Alistair, the city administrator in Chapter 2, end up wasting years in psychotherapy because their underlying problem is never addressed.

Patients who abuse mind/emotion-altering substances (alcohol, prescription or illegal drugs, etc.) don't usually reveal this information to their psychotherapists on their own. But because you are reading this book, this probably means you are serious about getting better. You don't want to waste your time and money on ineffective, pointless therapy. Therefore, I want to ask you to disclose any information about substance use or abuse to a psychotherapist during the first session, even if he *doesn't* ask you questions about it. You may have one too many glasses of wine every evening than you would want to admit, or you may be overusing sleeping pills or painkillers; whatever the issue, therapy can't begin until treatment for substance abuse is under way. So give your therapist the information he needs to do his job right.

If you do have substance abuse issues, a responsible therapist will refer you to an addiction specialist or treatment program. If he doesn't, it is probably because he hasn't had the training to recognize that serious abuse or addiction to substances can cause symptoms of emotional and mental illness in a patient, including such common symptoms as anxiety and depression. Although I wish this weren't the case, it is up to you, the patient, to get the help you need if a psychotherapist isn't properly directing you. If you aren't having success with a general psychotherapist regarding any substance abuse issues, I recommend that you seek out an addiction specialist (preferably a co-occurring disorder specialist) who can help you with both emotional problems and chemical dependency or refer you to a treatment program and group therapy, if that is indicated.

After (or possibly before) your drug and alcohol history, the therapist will ask you a series of questions about your emotional and mental health. These will be extensive, and will include questions about whether or not you have been treated for a mental health problem in the past, as well as numerous related details, including a description of the onset of your problems, how severely they affect you, and if you have been taking medication or have been hospitalized. These questions will help the therapist determine how serious your issues are and if their presence indicates you could be a threat to yourself or others.

Medical History

The next set of questions the therapist should ask you will concern your physical health. If you are depressed and lacking energy, for example, he may ask if you have had your thyroid or blood sugar tested. If you say no, he may recommend that you get a comprehensive medical exam in the near future.

He should feel certain that your problems are psychological or psychiatric in origin, not related to a medical condition. The converse is also possible; sometimes a psychological or psychiatric problem could be misinterpreted as stemming from a medical cause.

I feel very strongly that if a therapist does not begin with a written biopsychosocial evaluation during your very first session (it could possibly take him up to two sessions or, in rare cases, even longer to complete the initial evaluation), you should ask him in a clear and direct manner to give you one. If his answer is that he doesn't "believe" in them, or that it isn't part of his clinical philosophy, then you should tell him you prefer to see a therapist who believes in their importance. No therapist can understand the larger picture (as well as the salient details) of a person's life without a detailed evaluation. He won't be able to make a diagnosis, and he certainly won't be able to make a plan for your treatment.

Detailed Notes

In addition to taking notes during your sessions, your therapist should also make notes as soon as possible afterward, when he is able to focus intently. I have heard from more than a handful of patients that it seems to them that many therapists just don't bother to take notes during sessions, but I can't emphasize enough the importance of note-taking. Your family, spouse, and friends don't need to take notes about you because they've had years to get to know you, and you're probably not paying them to treat you for emotional problems anyway. It is your therapist's job to cut to the chase and get to know you in a far shorter period of time.

The biopsychosocial evaluation and subsequent session notes are also important because they can refresh (or replace, in some cases) a therapist's memory. If he has written notes, he will be able to review your case whenever he needs to. The great Freudians of yesteryear used to train themselves to memorize enormous amounts of detail about each patient—today's therapists aren't trained to do this.

Don't waste your time and money—only work with a therapist who is going to put a serious effort into helping you get better, one who cares enough to do the groundwork. Sitting back and merely listening to you talk about your life is not what a therapist should be doing with your time and money.

Your First Session and Follow-up

Here is how I generally conduct a first session. First, I have a ten- or fifteen-minute discussion with a patient to briefly get to know him, then tell him that I want to ask him some specific questions (the evaluation) that can help me get to know and understand his problems. I tell him that his answers can help us work together on a plan of action (the treatment plan) that will help ameliorate those problems. I tell him that without this information, I would be unable to understand the context for the therapy and would not be able to develop a structure for the treatment. I strongly believe that the structural process of therapy has to be transparent and basically understood by the patient.

Before your session ends, your therapist will most likely ask you if you want to make another appointment. If you feel things went well, go ahead. I do recommend, though, that you first ask the therapist how your treatment will be structured in terms of (1) the frequency of sessions and (2) the amount of time needed to complete a course of treatment.

Though he may not have all the answers during the very first session (it might take him two or three times to give you more concrete answers), he should be able to give you a very general idea about how often he thinks he will need to see you and about how long therapy will take. I find that it helps alleviate anxiety if a patient can get some real clarity during the very first session; so if the patient agrees, I try to schedule a lengthier first session that is anywhere from one and a half to two hours long. This way I can do a thorough initial evaluation as well as give the patient an overview of the structure of the course of his therapy.

Your therapist will be able to be more explicit in future sessions once he gets to know you better, and when your treatment plan has begun to be developed. If you aren't sure you want to make another appointment, tell him you would rather think about it and get back to him. After only one session, he shouldn't pressure you in any way to make an appointment. Later on, in another session or two, when he wants to ensure that you are committed to the process and not going to begin a clinical course of treatment and drop out, he may ask you to make a commitment to regular sessions.

How do therapists really know what clinical course of treatment to follow? In the *Diagnostic and Statistical Manual of Mental Disorders* (DSM-IV-TR), the bible of mental health for all psychotherapists, algorithms are given. These are based on a patient's answers to the initial evaluation. The algorithms—frequently referred to as "decision trees"—guide therapists and help them rule in or out various disorders. Of course, experienced therapists may not need to refer to the manual all the time. Once the therapist has a good idea what the problem is, he will be able to decide on a course of treatment.

We suggest that you don't rely on any therapist to perform every single course of action we recommend in this book. No one is perfect, and your therapist may forget something or make an error or have a different approach in some particulars. This is why you must rely on yourself to make sure you are getting the best treatment possible. Interestingly, advocating for yourself can actually be an important part of the therapeutic process. Not only will this book help you know what to look for in a therapist, it will also help you develop the confidence you need to ask your therapist to step up to the plate in those areas where he may not be making as great an effort as he should. We want to help you get excellent treatment that is worth your investment in time and money.

Below you will find two checklists: the first one will help you make sure that you have been given a thorough evaluation, while the second will help you evaluate your first session with your therapist.

Biopsychosocial History/Evaluation Checklist

Make sure that *at least* the following topics are included:

❑ 1. Identifying data/demographic data (social security number, date of birth, sex, race, emergency contact information, living situation)

❑ 2. Alcohol and drug history (including over-the-counter and prescription medications, herbal or nutritional remedies, and illegal drugs and alcohol; how drugs are administered; frequency of use; age first used; date last used; progression of use; withdrawal symptoms; history of treatment programs/hospitalizations; symptoms and complications of alcohol and drug history)

❑ 3. Mental health history (including medication history and compliance, allergies to medications, history of treatment programs/ hospitalizations, and symptoms and complications of that history, including harm to self or others)

❑ 4. Medical history (including medication history and compliance, allergies to medications, hospitalizations, chronic and/or life-threatening illnesses, and symptoms and past and current complications of that history)

❑ 5. Other topics (sexual history, educational history, vocational history, financial history, legal history, social history, family/significant other, gambling history, nicotine history, eating disorders, spirituality, leisure, military history)

❑ 6. Reason for seeking treatment

❑ 7. Questions specific to present stage of life (childhood, adolescence, geriatric, etc., as needed)

Patient's Own Therapist Evaluation Worksheet

Now is the time to begin getting in touch with your thoughts and feelings about therapy and any therapist you are considering working with. This worksheet will help you evaluate a therapist.

(Check Yes or No)

1. The therapist's office was reasonably comfortable and clean.
   - ○ Yes, the office was comfortable and clean.
   - ○ No, the office was not comfortable and clean.

2. The therapist was punctual, or, if not, let me know he was running late with an urgent situation.
   - ○ Yes, the therapist was punctual.
   - ○ No, he was not punctual.

3. The therapist maintained healthy physical boundaries and did not use inappropriate touch.
   - ○ Yes, the therapist maintained healthy physical boundaries and did *not* use inappropriate touch.
   - ○ No, the therapist didn't maintain healthy physical boundaries and touched me inappropriately.

4. The therapist was forthcoming when (if) I asked to see his credentials.
   - ○ Yes, he showed me his credentials when asked.
   - ○ No, he did not show me his credentials when asked.

5. The therapist clearly answered any questions I had about his credentials or referred me to resources that could help me understand.
   - ○ Yes, he answered my questions about credentials.
   - ○ No, he didn't answer my questions about credentials.

6. The therapist seemed to be caring and concerned about me.
   - ○ Yes, he seemed to be caring and concerned.
   - ○ No, he did not seem to be caring and concerned.

7. The therapist asked a lot of questions during my first visit.
   - ○ Yes, he asked a lot of questions.

O No, he did not ask a lot of questions.

8. The therapist listened carefully to my answers.
   O Yes, he listened carefully to my answers.
   O No, he did not listen carefully to my answers.

9. The therapist did a biopsychosocial evaluation and wrote down my answers. (In certain cases this might take a couple of visits to complete, but it should be begun during the first session.)
   O Yes, he did an evaluation and wrote down my answers.
   O No, he did not do an evaluation.

10. The therapist asked me basic questions about who I am, questions about my mental health, questions about substance abuse, and questions about my physical health. (This might take a couple of visits to complete.)
    O Yes, he asked about my mental and physical health and if I use or abuse drugs or alcohol.
    O No, he did not ask me about my mental and physical health and if I use or abuse drugs or alcohol.

11. The therapist answered my questions in a detailed manner about what would happen next if I chose to continue therapy with him.
    O Yes, he answered my questions. O No, he did not answer my questions.

12. The therapist did not pressure me to make another appointment with him.
    O Yes, he did not pressure me. O No, he pressured me.

13. The balance of talking and listening during my session was comfortable for me.
    O Yes, it was. O No, it was not.

14. Overall I feel comfortable with this therapist and think that he/she can help me.
    O Yes, I feel comfortable with this therapist.
    O No, I do not feel comfortable with this therapist.

Chapter 5

DEVELOPING A TREATMENT PLAN: YOUR MAP TO SUCCESS

On a journey of a hundred miles, ninety is but half way.

—CHINESE PROVERB

A *treatment plan* is a written plan created by a therapist and patient that is used as a guide to how therapy should ideally proceed in order to address clinical and any other relevant life issues. It is central to effective therapy. A few years ago we published an article in a weekly newspaper on the use of treatment plans in psychotherapy. At the time I believed that the use of treatment plans was ubiquitous—after all, how could therapy proceed without a plan? There must be a written understanding and statement of the patient's problems, a statement of the therapeutic goals, and a well-structured strategy of how to alleviate the problems and achieve the goals. Seems obvious, right?

In the article I primarily aimed at explaining the reasons why it was worthwhile for therapists to use valuable session time writing a treatment plan. It does take a certain amount of time to build a good plan, and I wanted patients to know why this was time well spent and why they shouldn't try to

e

rush through the process. I tried to convey that the development of a treatment plan is yet another example of taking the longer-shorter path—without a plan, therapy would be a hit-or-miss affair and consequently take much more time in the long run.

I also had another (what I thought of as minor) reason to write the article. Based on what I had been hearing, it seemed that not all therapists were putting as much effort into treatment plans as they should. Some patients mentioned (to my colleagues as well as to me) that they hadn't received written plans, though plans had been verbalized on occasion. I wanted patients to understand the importance of having a *written* plan that both the therapist and patient agreed to. I also wanted to help patients learn how to advocate for themselves in this matter. Therefore, the article stated that a well-developed, written treatment plan was a priority.

The response to the article took me completely by surprise. Within a couple of days of publication, dozens of patients and their families phoned and e-mailed me. Their stories were similar. Not only did they not know about the centrality of treatment plans to treatment, they didn't even know such a thing as a treatment plan existed. The majority of people who phoned me said that they had never even heard of them until they read the article. Their therapists had just not bothered to mention treatment plans at all.

Georgia: Demanding a Treatment Plan

One woman, Georgia, a frustrated mom, called to share her experience. Her son Mike had been in treatment for nearly four years with the same therapist. Mike had behavioral issues, learning challenges, and was mildly depressed. After reading my article and learning about the seminal importance of a treatment plan, Georgia, a caring mom, who had been suspicious for a while about the efficacy of her son's therapy, scheduled an appointment with the therapist for herself. When she got there, she handed him the article and asked him to show her Mike's treatment plan. He hemmed and hawed and finally said he didn't "believe in working with treatment plans."

Georgia explained, "He shuffled around the papers on his desk and wouldn't look me in the eye." She was livid. "You have been treating my son for a host of problems for four years, and you don't have a plan for his treatment? Week after week I have been bringing him here and he has only become more and more depressed. You kept assuring me he was making progress. How could he be making progress if you don't even know what his goals should be, let alone have a plan on how to achieve them?" I think Georgia would have made a great lawyer!

She also told me that the therapist responded to her admittedly angry tirade by telling her that she had an anger management problem. He recommended that she get therapy. Ha. The therapist's response was a classic dodge—if you offer sincere, relevant criticisms of him, you are the one with the problem.

Don't let this happen to you. I recommend that if by the middle of your second session your therapist hasn't started to work on a treatment plan with you, you should directly ask, "When will we get to work on my written treatment plan?" This should spur him to take action.

I can only guess why some therapists are not doing the necessary basics of therapy, such as performing thorough evaluations and writing treatment plans. Perhaps therapists in private practice who do not accept insurance (and therefore are not forced to submit treatment plans to supervisors, insurance companies, and HMOs) may become lax in their observance of protocol. A little knowledge and assertiveness on your part will hopefully convince a lax therapist to be more responsible.

Building a treatment plan is work. It holds the therapist (as well as the patient) accountable for meeting the goals it contains. Since there are no regulating agencies that oversee individual therapy sessions, I am sorry to say that in many instances a therapist can get away with not writing a treatment plan.

Today, most therapists in private practice have trained in clinics or hospitals, or work in one full- or part-time, and have a part-time private practice as well. Each and every case in a clinic or hospital must have a written treatment plan, so it is reasonable to assume that *all* therapists are aware of the necessity of creating one. Try Googling "psychotherapy treatment plan." There are nearly half a million links. Certainly this is not an esoteric treatment tool no one has ever heard of.

Insurance Company Rationale

Why do you think HMOs and insurance companies require therapists to submit treatment plans if they want to be paid? It's not only because a treatment plan shows the insurance company that realistic and measurable goals have been set and that a treatment plan is written evidence that actual work is being done by the therapist, but it's also because insurance companies know that it is simply good therapy—having a treatment plan helps patients get better faster. And the sooner a patient gets well and the longer his recovery lasts, the less money the insurance company will have to pay out in the long run.

It is cost-effective for the HMOs and insurance companies to have an agent review the treatment plan before they approve payment. It makes both financial and clinical sense for therapy to have a beginning, middle, and most important, an end. The insurance companies don't want to keep paying for treatment without an end in sight. They want to see that the money will be/was used to good effect. Only a treatment plan (and the discharge plan, which occurs at the end of therapy) can provide that information. In fact, when they first started setting standards and limits, insurance companies hired teams of psychotherapy professionals to set the standards for psychotherapy reimbursements. These professionals determined that the treatment plan is indispensable to therapy (and to the insurance companies), because without it, none of the clinical work can be planned, measured, or assessed. Today the most effective therapists use this important treatment tool whether they take insurance or not. As you read more about what good therapy involves, you will understand why we keep stressing and restressing the pivotal role treatment plans should have in your treatment.

Mapping Therapy: How a Treatment Plan Is Built

Once your evaluation is completed, the individualized treatment plan can begin to be developed. The treatment plan is derived from the findings of the evaluation and could take up to a few sessions to be written up. The maximum amount of time it should take to write a fully developed (though open to changes) plan is thirty days, though a plan should at least be started during your second visit. Depending on the complexity of your reasons for seeking therapy, your therapist may need to take more time to fully begin to understand what issues exist, what issues you want to/are ready to address, and how to address them. And don't forget—your own input is integral to developing an appropriate plan.

In the case of an individual under the age of eighteen, a parent will give input into the creation of, as well as regularly review, the treatment plan, but in the vast majority of adult therapy cases, the therapist should always work together directly with the patient.

As you begin to work together on your treatment plan, your therapist will usually write on paper or type into a computer while you and he develop the contents. As we mentioned in Chapter 4, your therapist should take notes during all your sessions, not just while you are building your treatment plan. Some therapists may prefer to record sessions on tape and write up everything afterward, and may ask for your permission to do so. Since many patients are not comfortable with this, most therapists don't even bother to ask and just write notes during the session.

The treatment plan should always be written out—not tucked away in the therapist's mind—and you should be given your own copy of it. You should have time to review the treatment plan, discuss changes you might want to make to the plan with your therapist, and then sign and date it if you approve it. Your therapist, too, should sign the plan. If at any point the plan needs to be modified, it should be done in writing, and you and the therapist should write your initials next to the amendment.

No. 1: Problem Statement

A treatment plan is like a personalized map of your therapy. The therapist can be thought of as your GPS system, guiding you step-by-step. First, you have to know your starting point. Knowing where you are starting out is defined in the *problem statement*, which is based (at least initially) on the evaluation.

The therapist should share his findings from the evaluation with you. Your individualized treatment plan will begin with a summary of your problems as they are presented in the evaluation (as well as in any subsequent conversations). It will be written in the form of a problem statement or statements. These problem statements might read something like: "Jennifer dropped out of school because of failing grades," or "Mark exhibits signs of depression," or "Tyler is angry and oppositional when speaking to his wife and children."

Most people will have more than one problem, and generally between two and eight problems are listed in the problem statements section. That doesn't mean that all these problems will be addressed during the course of therapy; these statements are simply stating that the problems exist. Problem statements that are not relevant initially can be deferred to a later time when the time is right to address them.

No. 2: Treatment Goal(s)

Treatment goals are the patient's clinical (and sometimes life) goals as described in the treatment plan. You and your therapist have to know where you are going in order to get there! Therapy that meanders on without a clearly defined destination (and perhaps a couple of important pit stops on the way) reminds me of a scene in an old movie where the distraught hero jumps into a cab. "Where're you going, buddy?" asks the cabbie. Our hero says, "Nowhere in particular. Just drive." That's a fine idea if you are a hero in a black-and-white movie trying to forget your broken heart, but a terrible idea if you are in therapy. *Your primary destination must be the completion of your treatment goal(s).*

Your own input is crucial here. Generally speaking, your treatment goals are the opposite of your problem statements. But they may deviate from that format based on your own personal input. Remember our imaginary patient Jennifer and her problem statement: "Jennifer dropped out of school because of failing grades." Her treatment goal might be something like this: "Jennifer wants to return to school and continue her studies." Or, if she indicates there are other options she wants to consider, something like this: "Jennifer wants to reevaluate her educational goals and decide if she wants to return to school or focus more on her music."

On the other hand, Mark, who is suffering from depression, might have a goal that states: "Mark will be free from the signs and symptoms of depression." And Tyler, who is unable to control his aggression, might have as his goal: "Tyler will learn how to communicate in a nonthreatening manner."

No. 3: Therapist's Objectives

So how will Jennifer, Mark, Tyler, and you get to your destinations? In large part, you'll get there with the guidance and support of your therapist. In addition to his caring nature, your therapist will have several methods at his disposal to help you chart your route to achieve your treatment goals. The courses of action that your therapist takes in order to help you achieve your goals are known as *objectives*. These objectives may even describe the specific *interventions* (another term for psychotherapeutic techniques or methods that begin the healing process) or techniques the therapist will use.

In this section of your treatment plan, your therapist will write down what he is going to do to help you achieve your goals. For example, concerning Mark, Dr. Gold, his therapist, might write down objectives like this:

1. Help Mark understand and talk about what the signs and symptoms of depression are.
2. Help Mark identify and talk about three external factors that trigger his depression.
3. Help Mark identify and talk about three internal factors that trigger his depression.
4. Teach Mark proven methods to help alleviate the signs and symptoms of depression that he is experiencing.

Usually one or two of the therapist's treatment objectives are enough to focus on in the beginning. Your therapist may introduce objectives gradually instead of all at once.

No. 4: Patient's Objectives

If the therapist is the GPS system, you are the driver. Ultimately, you have control over where you are going emotionally and how you get there. Your therapist shouldn't force you to press the gas pedal if your internal traffic light is red, or turn right when your heart says to go straight.

With a therapist who is trustworthy, competent, and caring, you will find that his guidance will be in sync or just slightly ahead of your readiness to proceed, though he may push or prod occasionally. He might even be slightly behind. However, your therapist must be largely in tune with or aware of your pace and adjust his objectives accordingly.

Including your own objectives in the treatment plan is an important way to keep reminding yourself that you are the driver. Your own treatment objectives, when written down, will most likely mirror your therapist's. For example, Mark's objectives might look something like this:

1. Mark will identify and talk about what the signs and symptoms of his depression are.
2. Mark will identify and describe three external situations that trigger his depression.
3. Mark will identify and describe three internal situations that trigger his depression.

4. Mark will learn and use proven method(s) he is learning from his therapist and will report back in each session how these methods have been employed, as well as describe their effectiveness.

Not all patient objectives will be this specific, but developing an understanding of specific, even seemingly minute goals can help you develop a supportive structure in which to work. *Identifying and working toward achieving tangible, achievable goals is one of the most important aspects of therapy.*

If your therapist or you believe that your goals are difficult to specify or measure (and this may certainly be the case), he must work with you to describe these goals in as material and functional a way as possible. In other words, he must help you make intangible goals more tangible. For example, if your goal is to develop a better awareness of your feelings, your therapist should help you define the terms "awareness" and "feelings," explain why this goal is important and relevant to you, and make a very real plan describing the steps needed to accomplish it.

Setting and then methodically working to achieve your goals will do more than merely help you solve the particular problems you are addressing. The process itself will teach you (1) how to focus on what is important to you in many areas of your life and (2) how to do things step-by-step. Applying these two important skills in other areas of your life outside of therapy will enable you to have a greater understanding of *all* your life goals. This will help you get to know yourself and help you develop the inner strength to achieve more in your life.

Denise: Getting Off Track

Denise Ryan, an editor of a scholarly journal, is from Boston. She entered therapy in order to work on fighting the inertia she felt after her marriage ended. She wanted to find a new relationship and explore career options, but hesitated to make the effort because of the sadness the divorce triggered in her.

Therapy had helped her brother cope with some problems, so she thought she should give it a try. Lori, her newfound therapist, was personable and caring, but after only the most cursory evaluation didn't bother to create a treatment plan with Denise. After a few sessions, Lori began to ask Denise more and more questions about her childhood. Denise felt this was really going off track, but she still hesitated to confront her. Several months later Lori was telling Denise that she needed to work on her anger issues, and that the grief she felt over the breakup of her marriage was really disguised anger.

When Denise, a rather rigorously honest individual, expressed puzzlement at this proclamation, the therapist told her that Denise repeatedly mentioned her anger and even rage during their first couple of sessions and had specifically asked to work on these issues. Denise insisted she never said any such thing. She remembered specifically that she told Lori she was somewhat sad and disappointed, yet Lori kept on insisting that she did mention anger. Finally, after three more sessions spent in fruitless back-and-forth disagreement, Denise decided that she wanted to see another therapist. She came to a colleague of mine who, after a comprehensive evaluation, worked on a treatment plan with Denise that focused on addressing her lingering (though minor) sadness and her desire for a new career. Denise now had a written treatment plan. Both Denise and her new therapist were able, with quite a bit of accuracy, to remember why Denise entered therapy in the first place.

Surprising as it seems, these essential life skills are not often taught. Somehow people are expected to understand how to develop a life direction without having the process explained. Your treatment plan may be the first time in your life that you examine problems close-up and work on solving them in focused manner. Good therapy should be a map for life.

No. 5: Target Dates and Check-in

Target dates are the optimal dates by which one or more treatment goals should be assessed and/or achieved. Will you arrive at your destination next Tuesday or will you be on the road for a couple of months? Setting target dates is an essential part of your treatment plan.

The target dates you and your therapist set will probably correspond to both long- and short-term goals, with short-term goals having priority. Complex goals (like the alleviation of Mark's depression) can be broken down into manageable parts, and intermediate target dates can be set for each of these subgoals. Ninety days from the beginning of treatment is usually a standard target date many therapists are comfortable setting. But patients may be able to resolve some issues in sixty or thirty days. I strongly recommend that initially you set at least one reasonable goal with a target date no more than thirty days from the beginning of treatment. In most cases this is enough time for you to evaluate whether or not you can work comfortably with a particular therapist. By holding the therapist—and yourself— accountable to achieve a specific goal in a reasonable, but short time frame, you will help create the setting in which highly focused and effective therapy can take place.

During each session, your therapist and you should take some time, even just a few minutes, to review the part of the treatment plan you are currently working on. Together you will evaluate your progress and measure it against your target dates. When you complete a goal, it can be noted on your treatment plan that the goal was achieved. Also, your therapist should review your other goals with you occasionally. This is important because some of the initial treatment goals you set may no longer be relevant or desirable. If this is the case, you may amend your goals. Anytime you and your therapist agree that there should be amendments to your treatment plan, they should be noted (see No. 9).

If your therapist isn't as proactive as I've outlined earlier, or even if he is, you really need to take responsibility for monitoring the progress of your therapy. Don't hesitate to ask your therapist for feedback on your progress. How does he think you are doing? See if his sense of your progress matches your own perceptions; if they don't, you will need to talk about this and decide what should be done about it.

For example, let's return to Mark's story and discuss two possible outcomes. After three months of therapy, Mark wasn't feeling that his depression was much better. He still found himself oversleeping and not eating regularly. However, Dr. Gold felt that Mark had made dramatic improvements. He reminded Mark that before therapy, he was reclusive and only left his house to go to work. Now Mark was going out to mow the lawn, and recently even went out for pizza with an old friend. Because Dr. Gold pointed out Mark's achievements, Mark realized that he really was making improvements, and this recognition spurred him on to greater success.

In an alternate telling of Mark's story, Mark believes he is making pretty good progress, but Dr. Gold says, "Hold on a moment. Yes, you are making some progress, but it isn't as much as you seem to believe. Let's talk about that." All types of scenarios can play out—you and your therapist will naturally have some difference of opinion about how you are doing. It doesn't necessarily mean that your viewpoints are incompatible.

However, if your therapist and you have widely divergent viewpoints on your progress, this can be a red flag. It is even possible that an unethical therapist might prey upon your vulnerabilities by telling you that you are sicker than you are or even "helping" you create imaginary illnesses or situations by triggering upsetting memories. Or you might feel that your problem is extremely overwhelming, and an inexperienced therapist might make light of potential dangerous symptoms. Basically, by checking in with yourself and with your therapist about your progress and examining the information you gleaned during this check-in, you can assess how things are going. By reviewing and assessing the progress you have made so far and comparing it to your set goals and target dates, you should get a reasonable idea of how therapy is progressing.

No. 6: Partners in Therapy

Everyone in your life—from your boss, to your mom, to your husband— is potentially a part of your therapy. This doesn't mean they have to come to sessions with you; in fact, it doesn't mean they even have to know you are in therapy! What it does mean is that because so much of therapy is about relationships, how you participate in these relationships is a subject that will most likely come up time and again.

Of course, there may be times when a spouse or parent could help you better achieve your goals if they do sit in on a session with you. Or specific relationships themselves might be an integral part of your reason for being in therapy. If that is the case, the therapist may recommend that one or more of your family members join you in therapy for one or more sessions. This should be discussed and written down in your treatment plan.

For example, Mark moved back home after college. He felt that the stress of living with his parents made him more depressed. Although he contributed to the household bills and chores as any responsible adult would, his parents still set strict limits on Mark's activities. Mark felt this to be demeaning. Dr. Gold had initially decided that Mark should work on his depression in individual therapy, but he wrote a note in the treatment plan that after sixty days had passed, Mark and he would revisit the idea of bringing one or both parents in for a session.

At that point both Mark and Dr. Gold agreed that he had made enough progress that he could comfortably invite both parents to a session. Mark's parents genuinely wanted their son to be strong enough to move forward (and out!). They were very willing to come to a session or two. With Dr. Gold's help, Mark was able to tell his parents that he wanted to be free to make his own mistakes and learn from them. Mark was so pleased with the reasonable compromise he and his parents negotiated with Dr. Gold's help that he felt much happier and stronger than he had in a long time. His parents were true partners in therapy, and Dr. Gold helped Mark make the most of the partnership.

Of course, sometimes, for any number of reasons, those invited to participate in your therapy session may not want to participate. They might believe you have unresolved anger toward them and fear a confrontation, or they don't feel that their point of view will be heard. Or they may simply feel that you are the one with the problem and not them. Some people might just not feel comfortable with the idea of therapy and are afraid of the outcome. There are many reasons significant others in your life might not want to join you in a session. Sometimes they will come to therapy sessions for reasons that might not be very productive. They might come in order to show that they are right and you are wrong, and that any problems in the relationship are because of you.

No one can be forced to participate in therapy unless by court order. If the relationship is highly contentious, yet is an important relationship in your life, you may have to accept the fact that for now that person won't participate. In this case your therapist should help you develop coping skills that can carry you through the relationship until it is ready to become "unstuck."

Other, more impersonal partners in therapy could include an employer, a spiritual advisor, a medical doctor, or another type of therapist. These people, while usually on the peripheral of your personal life, are nonetheless often an important part of your life. The ways in which they can partner in your therapy are numerous. For example, your employer could be asked to give you extra time off to accomplish therapeutic goals. You may want to give your therapist permission to talk about your situation with your spiritual advisor or have a different reason for another person's involvement.

No. 7: Recommendations

Partners and recommendations are very closely related. Sometimes, in addition to your therapist, working with other professionals or types of therapies or activities can help you achieve your therapy goals. Your therapist might recommend you schedule additional appointments with other professionals that you are already seeing, or might even recommend you seek the services of new ones. He might suggest that your current medical doctor give you a specific medical test or possibly prescribe a medication. Or your psychotherapist could recommend you see a psychiatrist.

He might believe that social services such as government jobs programs could help you improve a situation you are struggling with. He might recommend you see a social worker who specializes in a particular area of concern. He might recommend that you attend *group psychotherapy* or advanced group psychotherapy, in which a group of patients participate, facilitated by one or more therapists, that makes use of a variety of techniques. Advanced group psychotherapy makes use of highly detailed and refined techniques and is extremely effective in helping resolve many deep-seated issues that conventional group psychotherapy or *individual psychotherapy*—the psychotherapeutic treatment of an individual by a therapist on a one-on-one basis—cannot. For example, *psychodrama,* developed in 1942 by Jacob L. Moreno, MD, is a powerful advanced group therapy technique that is particularly effective at helping patients learn and practice new emotional and behavioral skills in a safe, supportive setting. It is at once complex and refined, and several techniques, especially role playing, are used to bring about profound insights and positive changes in the participating patients. For a basic description of psychodrama see http://www.asgpp.org/html/psychodrama.html.

Your therapist could suggest you attend 12-step meetings, such as those offered by Alcoholics Anonymous (AA), or attend an outpatient substance abuse treatment program. The 12-step formula is used by individuals in their recovery from addiction and other dysfunctional behavior. Today there are many versions of the 12 steps, but the original can be found in the AA Big Book, which can be found online at http://www.aa.org/bbonline/.

Your therapist may even recommend that you take an art class, join a gym, or try a movement or bodywork program. All of these and many more potential partners and recommendations should be discussed as needed and made a part of your treatment plan. The recommendations should be part of the support system designed to resolve your problems and should take into account your unique strengths, needs, abilities, and preferences.

No. 8: Schedule of Services

An outline of the recommended frequency (and dates and times) of individual therapy sessions, as well as any schedules of other therapies or activities that might help you resolve your problems, should all be part of your treatment plan. Although the actual frequency of therapy sessions and other activities will most likely be adjusted as you progress, it is important that a schedule is committed to at first.

No. 9: Amendments and Changes

As your therapist gets to know you, and as you get to know yourself and get to know what therapy can do for you, you will find that your treatment plan will require slight amendments or occasionally dramatic changes. Goals may morph and become simpler or more complex. The need for frequent therapy sessions may decrease or increase. Some parts of your treatment plan may need to be completely deleted or put on hold to be revisited at a later date. In any of these instances, it is important for the changes to be noted and even initialed by you and your therapist. By indicating changes and making sure you both understand and have witnessed the changes, misunderstandings can be avoided.

No. 10: Other Sections

Other sections in your treatment plan may include descriptions of the ways in which various other professional or government services are coordinated (for example, if you were referred by the criminal justice system, how would this fact be incorporated into your plan?), descriptions of how services with your significant others would actually be coordinated, procedures for the structure of various care services, and so on.

Your Treatment Plan Checklist

Review this checklist before and after your second therapy session and compare it to your existing treatment plan. Your treatment plan may contain other elements not listed here. It might even call the components by different names, but the following essentials should be present in some form.

Think: What is causing difficulty in my life?

❏ 1. Problem statement: This statement (or statements) describes your problem or problems based on the evidence presented in the evaluation. Life areas that will form part of the evaluation and may form a problem statement include, but are not limited to, family and interpersonal relationships, professional relationships, daily living skills, legal problems, education, vocation, employment, social and leisure, sexuality, domestic violence, medical, health, nutrition, housing, spirituality, and so on.

Think: Where (who, what) do I want to be?

❏ 2. Treatment goal: This goal (or goals) describes the outcome both you and the therapist think will indicate success. The treatment goal must also be achievable. It is usually the opposite of the problem statement, but not always. It should also be a brief and concise statement of a general condition and should be forward-looking. It should be easy to infer from reading it that this goal intends to help you attain something better.

Think: How is my therapist going to help me get there?

❏ 3. Therapist objectives: These will be a list of techniques, methods, and/or descriptions of specific steps that the therapist will take to help you achieve your treatment goal. They must be concrete and measurable. These are the individual steps toward achieving the goal.

Think: How am I going to help myself get there?

❏ 4. Patient objectives: These will be a list of the patient's planned steps, actions, and objectives, which will most likely mirror the therapist's objectives. They must be concrete and measurable. These should easily be recognizable as being the individual steps needed to achieve the treatment goal. They should help you think "How am I going to get there?"

Think: When am I going to get there?

❑ 5. Target dates: These will be dates by which you and your therapist can expect to see measurable progress with one or more of your goals. At least one of your target dates should be set for thirty days, though you may have longer-term targets as well.

Think: Who else is part of my journey?

❑ 6. Partners in therapy: This will be a list of potential partners in your therapy and may include those who will come to sessions with you, as well as those who will not.

Think: Who else and what other activities will help me get there?

❑ 7. Recommendations: This will be a list of recommendations to get the help of other professionals, including those currently working with you and/or those whose help may be solicited now or in the future.

❑ 8. Schedule/frequency of services: This might include group, individual, family, psychiatric, psychological, occupational therapy, and integrated programs of therapies and activities to resolve the problem that incorporate the unique strengths, needs, abilities, and preferences of the patient.

Think: What changes may be necessary to make along the way?

❑ 9. Amendment/changes section: Discuss and list any revisions you have concerning the objectives, goals, partners, recommendations, and so on, as you regularly review your treatment plan.

Think: What other procedures will be put in place to facilitate my treatment?

❑ 10. Other: Other procedures, mechanisms for coordination of multiple services, other sections necessary to your individual treatment plan, and so on.

Using Your Treatment Plan for Success

❑ 1. Do you have a written treatment plan that you participated in creating together with your therapist?

❑ 2. Does it contain all the parts listed in the treatment plan checklist above?

❑ 3. Do you understand all the parts of the treatment plan?

❑ 4. Do you and your therapist review the treatment plan and discuss how therapy is progressing, at least briefly, during every session, or at least during every other session?

Chapter 6

Great Expectations:
What Good Therapy Looks,
Sounds, and Feels Like

It is a bad plan that admits of no modification.

—Publilius Syrus

Although the development of your treatment plan (and the contents of your evaluation, which will also be updated throughout therapy as your therapist learns more about you) will continue in some measure over the course of therapy, the first usable version should be completed in, at most, a couple of sessions. This treatment plan will become a springboard for the work that needs to be done in subsequent sessions and will often be among the first items addressed at these sessions.

Your therapist will usually begin a session by either (1) asking you friendly, open-ended questions about your day and/or about the time period that has elapsed since your last session and (2) briefly (or more lengthily, as needed) reviewing your treatment plan and using it as a jumping-off point from which to discuss your progress, reviewing sections of the plan that need attention or changing sections of the plan that need amending.

Friendly and Open-ended Questions

By asking friendly, open-ended questions about how you are doing, your therapist is aiming to strengthen his rapport with you, helping you to unwind and connect with him. If you and he "got down to work" right away, this abrupt beginning could set a clinical or formal tone to the session that could restrict the open exchange needed for good therapy to take place. In general, formality is about careful presentation of the self in more distant relationships, and for therapy to work, a patient needs to open up and reveal his more informal, natural self. Friendly discussion leads to more trust than a formal clinical tone, and trust is the backbone of the therapeutic relationship. Of course, even though the tone may be informal, a focused clinical objective is still going on, working in tandem with and fueled by, the more relaxed atmosphere.

The types of questions your therapist will ask you at the start of each visit will therefore be friendly, informal, general, and, most important, open-ended. Open-ended questions can't be answered with a simple yes or no. Yes/no answers might be fine on a history test, but they won't get you very far in therapy. By thinking through and then describing your experiences out loud, you are not only helping the therapist understand you, but also helping you understand yourself.

Process, Please

One line of open-ended questions your therapist may start with will be to ask you to describe recent events in your life. What you did during the interim between the last session and this one is an effective way to segue into the session. As you discuss these events, you and your therapist will *process* them, keeping in mind your treatment plan.

If you have spent any time around psychotherapists, you will have heard the term "process" mentioned often—perhaps too often. It is overused by enthusiastic believers who view any and every conversation as an opportunity to process information. Not all conversations are that complex in terms of needing to be processed. Really, all the term *process* means is to "talk out" or verbally examine the different angles of the events under discussion and your feelings, thoughts, and behaviors as they relate to these events and to your life in general. Together you and your therapist will explore, analyze, and come to understand your feelings, thoughts, and behaviors and generate solutions through the detailed discussion called processing. When you process a topic, you will also work on developing skills that can help you respond to similar events in the future. Processing the many happenings that make up your life can help you resolve to change for the better.

Laron: Identify and Apply

When Laron, a twenty-nine-year-old retail clerk, first came to see me he was having run-ins with his mother-in-law, Patricia. She babysat for his children daily, so she was almost always at his house when he came home from work. Our sessions often began with him saying, "My mother-in-law was driving me crazy all week."

In general, despite the enormous respect Laron had for his mother-in-law, a woman who had accomplished much in her life despite facing tremendous challenges, he was frustrated by her behavior. She persisted in trying to control her daughter Eve, Laron's wife. Patricia was brought up in a traditional Jamaican home where her own mother ruled the roost. "Patricia told Eve she shouldn't buy groceries at Shop Rite anymore but instead shop at Whole Foods because the produce was healthier and fresher. We can't afford to shop there on our salaries and she knows this. She is butting in and causing fights between Eve and me almost every day."

Laron came to therapy to work on other issues in his life. Because he viewed the problems with Patricia as minor, although annoying, we only discussed his relationship with Patricia briefly, devoting far more time to the other problems that had priority for him. Even so, after only two or three sessions Laron had developed a new, more emotionally descriptive vocabulary with which to describe his and Patricia's conflicts.

We began to talk about the differences between aggression, assertiveness, passivity, and passive-aggressiveness, and other emotions and behaviors related to confrontation. Laron was soon able to identify what was happening internally when he and Patricia had conflicts. He began to be able to employ the use of more subtle terms to describe his feelings and behaviors. "I got into another argument with my mother-in-law. I was trying to be assertive, but ended up being aggressive."

Laron wasn't yet able to manage his anger and aggression as much as he would have liked. We continued to use many of his confrontations as jumping-off points to discuss anger, fear, and other emotions in general. Laron wanted to better understand and manage his reactions in all areas of his life. During therapy sessions, as we examined the problem in some detail, I taught Laron the skills he needed to respond (act in a manner in which one's response is consciously managed to produce a positive effect in stressful situations) rather than react (act in an uncontrolled, often negative manner in response to a situation). He then began to apply the skills he learned in "real life," not just in my office.

You should answer the opening questions in any way you feel comfortable, bearing in mind that your answers may become a jumping-off point for processing. As I did with Laron, your therapist should encourage you to discuss your responses and reactions to various problems in your life. He should also help you identify what is going on inside you, and teach you skills that you can apply to various situations. You will not only gain a better understanding of your emotions, feelings, and behavior, but this understanding will help you make very real, positive changes in your life. When you share your successes during your sessions, your therapist will point out those achievements that demonstrate the progress you have made. He also might suggest you explore areas that you are hesitant to work on or find difficult making progress in.

Your therapist should have clinical justification for wanting to work on these particular areas with you. If you aren't sure that working on a specific problem makes sense to you, don't be afraid to ask him for the reason why he feels it will be beneficial to focus on it. His answer should be clear and make sense to you. Discussions about your successes, as well as areas where progress may be slow, will provide a bridge back to your treatment plan.

Reviewing Your Treatment Plan

Many, if not most, of the discussions you have during your sessions will directly relate to your treatment plan. Together you and your therapist will frame questions about your progress and assess how much of your therapy journey has been completed. Are you on the right road? Do you need to make a pit stop or detour? Are there potholes or is a bridge out? Perhaps you have found a shortcut and have almost reached your destination.

In other words: What objectives and goals have been completed? Does your treatment plan need to be amended or modified in any way? Are new approaches necessary in order to effect change? Are there other issues that have cropped up that might deserve more attention or even take precedence over what is called for in the treatment plan? Have you made such speedy progress that some protocols of your treatment plan are no longer necessary? Have you achieved your therapy goals? You may ask some or all of these questions over the course of your therapy. As you can see, it would be impossible to answer these crucial therapy questions without having a treatment plan to refer to.

Most philosophies of psychotherapy posit that therapy can only be effective if a written treatment plan is followed and amended, if necessary. I consider the treatment plan to be organic and alive—it shouldn't be too vague or general, but it should still be able to flex with you as you change and grow. As we have said before, the treatment plan also allows you and your therapist to see if you are progressing or not. *The treatment plan is how the clinical success of your therapy is measured.* That's why you must review it regularly during sessions, otherwise, your therapy will wander aimlessly, occasionally bumping into some successes, but more often just wasting time (and money). That is also why a competent therapist won't work without one.

There are, however, some psychoanalytic schools of therapy in which treatment plans aren't usually used. During this kind of therapy, the patient talks and talks with either few or no prompts from the therapist. Though, as mentioned previously, the general consensus is that psychoanalysis-type therapies aren't proven to work, they can conceivably work for highly intelligent, wealthy (psychoanalysis and its offshoots may last for years and cost a lot) individuals who are able to afford the luxury of taking many years and spending much money getting to know themselves. Notably, these therapies are *not* covered by insurance, and the lack of the use of an actual plan of treatment listing evidence-based protocols and measurable goals is why this is the case. It is unclear how many psychotherapists actually use long-term psychoanalytic techniques, so if this type of therapy isn't your cup of tea, be sure to ask your therapist during the phone interview, or in person, what his philosophies are; otherwise, you could end up in therapy for years.

Identifying Triggers

Let's return to Laron's story. Laron needed help handling Patricia's interference in his married life. He wanted—and appreciated—her babysitting help. In fact, he and his wife, Eve, regularly took her out to dinner and bought her small gifts in order to thank her. But he resented that Patricia told Eve how to run their home and raise their kids. Patricia's attempt to control Eve (and Laron, by default) made for many potentially explosive situations. Most of the time Laron managed to hold in his anger, though this always seemed to give him chest pains and headaches.

One of your therapist's jobs will be to help you identify *triggers*. A trigger is an internal or external mechanism that produces an emotion. Like the trigger on a gun, a psychological trigger is the mechanism that produces a reaction; in the case of a gun, an explosion. Triggers can be internal or external. Internal triggers are feelings, emotions, and thoughts; external triggers can be objects, events, places, situations, sensory stimulations (such as a smell or melody), or the words and actions of other people. Triggers are predictable in that if you aren't taught to manage your response to them, they will cause an immediate behavioral or emotional reaction.

One evening, shortly before Laron was going to leave for his therapy appointment with me, he and Eve put the kids to bed. While they were doing this, Patricia began to go through their refrigerator and pantry, making loud "tsk-tsking" sounds. She started writing on a notepad. Then she called Eve into the kitchen and began to show her out-of-date milk and moldy bread she had found in the fridge. In a loud voice she proceeded to explain her food-shopping system and why it was superior to the rather haphazard system Laron and Eve used.

Laron couldn't help overhearing. He hastily finished tucking in his youngest son and walked into the kitchen. "You know, Ma, it's not a big deal. So far the kids are all healthy, and we all get plenty to eat. So just throw out the old stuff, and I promise we'll buy fresh milk tomorrow."

Patricia immediately pounced. "You just go on to your *therapy*, Laron. I am Eve's mother, and I am the one who'll teach her how to run a house, not you. Don't worry about the house, just worry about your job. What goes on in this kitchen is really none of your business."

Laron began to get angry but managed to stop himself from losing his temper. In this instance, Patricia's actions and words were the triggers. These could easily have sent most people over the edge. Fortunately, at this point in therapy Laron had learned how to identify his particular triggers and not to allow his feelings to escalate. He already had worked on not allowing someone else—anyone else, even Patricia—to control his behavior. He took responsibility for his own responses. He wanted to make productive choices and therefore was able to take a step back. He didn't get mad. He didn't get even. He got assertive. Instead of exploding or becoming upset and developing chest pains, he took a deep breath and calmly told Patricia he "would have to think about what she said and decide at a later time what he was going to do about it, but now he was rushing out to his appointment."

The Disgruntlement Point

Laron told me that an image that worked particularly well for him was that of a teakettle being taken off the stove—this made the whistle stop. During a previous session I explained that the feeling of anger was like steam from a teakettle (patients might suggest an image themselves—in this case, Laron had a difficult time imagining an anger image, so I shared one of mine). If the steam hole (that makes the whistle) is blocked, the steam will still need to come out from somewhere. It might be the spaces between the lid and the kettle, or eventually, if there is no other release, the whole kettle might explode. If Laron couldn't manage to channel his anger in a positive manner, or dissipate it entirely by removing the boiling kettle from the heat source, his anger might explode into other areas of his life. His work, his marriage, his kids—all would have to deal with his dark moods. Also, as he had been doing earlier, Laron could end up holding in these unpleasant feelings, which caused him some very real physical symptoms, like chest pains and headaches.

The skills Laron and I worked on together in therapy helped him identify, manage, and dissipate his anger at or before the kettle exploded—in this case, the point when Laron felt most offended. I call this the *disgruntlement point*, the point at which an internal or external trigger becomes unmanageable and a behaviorally explosive reaction may occur. He now could pull that kettle off the fire whether he was triggered by Patricia, his boss, his kids, or anyone else he came into contact with. Soon he could apply the techniques he learned to other areas of his life. He also learned how to gain perspective on this situation and find new ways of looking at or reframing it.

Reframing the Situation

Your therapist should help you develop and apply the skills you need to *reframe* situations; that is, learn to look at events and relationships in your life in a more instructive way. Laron and I talked about how to view his situation with Patricia differently. He began to see that in certain areas Patricia was really not so bossy; it was primarily when it came to household tasks like shopping, cooking, and cleaning.

We talked about how important it was to listen and respond to the content of Patricia's message rather than react to the tone of her delivery. We talked about the possibility that those areas where Patricia was controlling were the only areas she felt confident about. He began to remind himself more often that she had good points and was even right, occasionally. He also began to think that far from undermining his masculinity, perhaps she was rather old-fashioned and believed that these areas were actually not "men's work" (despite the fact that both he and Eve worked outside the home, and that he often helped to clean, cook, and shop anyway). He saw that in Patricia's traditional worldview, she was actually complimenting him by telling him that he had "more important" things to attend to.

Real-life Consequences and Results

There are many real-life consequences to the behaviors that can arise from your feelings, emotions, and thoughts. Your therapist may encourage you to start by changing your feelings and thoughts, or he may ask you to work on changing your behavior first. In that case, your therapist will probably start by helping you reflect on all the various consequences of your not-so-positive behavior. Then he will help you respond to challenges with more beneficial behavior. He might help you get inspired by asking you to explore those times your behavior had very positive effects on your life.

As Laron's feelings toward Patricia began to change, and as he began to behave differently toward her, he found that her behavior toward him changed as well. She was by nature a generous person and even offered to help out with some of the cooking, stocking their freezer with stews and other nutritious food. Both Eve and Laron were relieved—neither really liked to cook, and there were some nights the kids had eaten cold cereal for dinner.

There are some surprising, far-reaching effects of good therapy. By helping you improve yourself, therapy can help you show others how to improve themselves. Once your behavior demonstrates greater levels of emotional maturity, the people you interact with will usually, either through direct discussion or by witnessing your role modeling, learn how to improve their behavior too. Psychotherapy can have many goals but understanding and improving the relationships in a patient's life is often a major goal. Therefore, the potential exists to change the world, one interpersonal network at a time.

Complexity and Growth

As you explore your current and past relationships you will, with guidance, begin to become more objective, less ego-centered, and better able to shed some of the more painful feelings that you may create or hold on to. Of course, when healing from trauma or coping with a severe mental illness or addiction, the information you learn in your sessions needs to be incorporated with many other skills and techniques you learn, too.

There are undeniably many levels of complexity of patients and problems. Laron was a very straightforward, intelligent, naturally easygoing young man whose personality, goals, and aspirations were not so complex. You might be more complex, and complexity can bring even greater opportunity for personal growth—and greater challenges.

For example, a colleague referred one of her patients, who I will call Samantha, to me. My colleague felt that Samantha would be best helped by working with someone who had experience with addiction, as she had been diagnosed several years earlier with a specific eating disorder related to addiction. Although her eating disorder was well under control, she now sought therapy to help with her vague, but constant feelings of fear and anxiety.

Samantha and her older sister were the owner-operators of a small interior design company. Samantha was the designer, and her sister ran the financial operations. They hired Rafael, a young, enthusiastic designer to help them with their work. Soon, client requests for Rafael's work eclipsed Samantha's own bookings. She consoled herself by saying she needed to concentrate on sales and purchases anyway, but she began to resent Rafael. Her resentment mushroomed. She secretly feared that her sister and the rest of her family would think Rafael was doing a better job than she was, though she had a difficult time articulating this. Samantha's fearful reactions to this and to numerous other relationships in her life compounded her anxiety.

Since her relationship with Rafael was far less overwhelming to Samantha than the problematic relationships she had with her family, we decided to tackle this problem first. Without exploring Samantha's troubled foundations too deeply, I suggested that perhaps the reason she resented Rafael was because she was comparing herself to him. Rather than recognizing and taking pride in the fact that she had organizational and entrepreneurial skills that Rafael did not have, she saw only her deficits. She reacted to his success by feeling threatened. In her worldview, someone else's achievements existed only in order to highlight her (perceived) lack of achievements. She bitterly resented Rafael's creative success, so much so that she even began to undermine him by complaining about him to her sister and clients and treating him disrespectfully. Naturally, this also began to undermine the stability of the company.

Together Samantha and I worked on understanding why she was reacting against her own best interests. In Samantha's case, we would have to eventually explore some aspects of her past, especially her family life where the roots of these issues could be found, but first we primarily concentrated on addressing problems she faced in the present. We also worked hard to help her develop the social skills she needed. Eventually she was able to apply the insights and solutions she had learned to many other situations in her life.

First, she had to become aware of some of the underlying reasons she resented Rafael and the apparently faulty ways of thinking that led her to do so. I mentioned to Samantha that perhaps Alcoholics Anonymous had a description for what she was doing: "Comparing your own insides with someone else's outsides," and that this comparison could only create a very uncomfortable feeling inside. By comparing herself to someone else in this manner,

Samantha left herself with only two real possibilities: either she was inferior to the other person or superior. If you see yourself as inferior to another, naturally that would feel unpleasant (unless, of course, you saw the person as a role model to be emulated); surprisingly, seeing yourself as superior also can create unpleasant feelings (and naturally will alienate others, as well).

Developing Awareness

I used various clinical techniques, including a very effective one called *motivational interviewing* (also used with Alistair from Chapter 2) to help Samantha martial her inner resources. The combination of techniques helped her develop awareness, maturity, and the ability to put her feelings in perspective.

Samantha: I am sick of Rafael. He is a real know-it-all. He better remember that he's lucky he still has his job.

Richard: What you are saying is that you feel you are being very gracious in allowing Rafael to continue to work for your company.

Samantha: That's right.

Richard: Let me ask you something, Samantha. What were the feelings and thoughts you were having just before you told me you were fed up with Rafael?

Samantha: Well, before I came here today Rafael was going on and on about color and light in design. He was acting like a know-it-all. I guess that's what I was thinking about while I was driving here.

Richard: You do have very good points, Samantha. Perhaps Rafael is overstepping his boundaries. Perhaps he is a bit too gung-ho. Perhaps you are right—he does think he knows more than you. But maybe there is a bit more to it than that. When he acts that way, he seems to trigger uncomfortable feelings in you. Maybe his behavior seems threatening to you.

Samantha: Yes.

Richard: So in some way it sounds like you perceive Rafael as being a threat to you.

Samantha: I didn't say that he is a threat. Well . . . I guess I feel like it sometimes. Actually, yes—that is exactly how it feels.

Richard: Of course, maybe it isn't as simple as that. Maybe his success in dealing with the other customers is what is so frustrating.

Samantha: Yeah. The customers and even my sister think he does it all. They don't know that I work hard, too.

Richard: So it feels to you as if his actions and behaviors are eclipsing you. They are noticing his successes, not yours.

Samantha (beginning to cry): Yes. They only see his success.

Richard: Let's look at this from another perspective, Samantha, because I think you aren't remembering all the hard work you do for your company and the successes you have had. Why don't you list what your contributions to the company are?

Samantha: Well, I do some design work, but mainly I put the finishing touches on Rafael's work. I also do almost all the sales and outreach to new clients. I manage the advertising and public relations. I manage relationships with all our suppliers. I attend all the trade shows and decide which trends the company should focus on. (*Samantha's list was too extensive to continue here.*)

As Samantha began to shift her awareness to the projects she was involved in and her own achievements, she also remembered that she was the one who hired Rafael in the first place, which she realized was much to her credit. Within a few weeks, she no longer felt she needed to be in the spotlight to be a success and eventually began to measure her success by her own inner guidelines.

Although it took several sessions for Samantha's resentment toward Rafael to begin to fade, she was eventually able to make the shift, and even became so appreciative of Rafael's contribution to the company that she gave him a promotion. The promotion made him even more visible to clients, but that was okay with Samantha—his success no longer threatened her. However, it took Samantha nearly a year to develop lasting self-esteem in other areas of her life, and several more months to work on some other issues. Laron had been able to effectively deal with his anger problems within a matter of months, and within six months he had completed therapy. Samantha needed about a year and a half.

The above examples illustrate just a couple of the reasons people come to therapy and how therapy can help them. There are, however, many kinds of problems that bring people to therapy. Each person's problems are unique, but generally fall into several general categories recognizable to a skilled therapist. When you and your therapist agree to address both the objectives and goals outlined in your treatment plan, as well as other important problems that come up, the work of therapy can take place. In addition to the discussions about events in your life, feelings, thoughts, emotions, and behaviors, your reactions to therapy itself can be a part of the therapy process.

The Inner Session

What is going on with a patient internally (the feelings and thoughts going on inside) right before, during, and after a session? I call this the *inner session*. On one level, there is tremendous energy being generated, although you might not always feel that way. Before a session you may feel excited, anxious, positive, negative, or have other strong feelings.

Sometimes, though, a patient will feel apathetic about therapy. Assuming the patient is working with a good therapist, and one who is right for him, the feelings of apathy could be a cover for feelings of anger and fear. Sometimes uncovering your problems and seeing yourself more objectively can be scary. You might unconsciously quash these uncomfortable feelings by feeling, or convincing yourself, that you feel apathetic.

If you find yourself feeling apathetic (or overly fearful, angry, or confused about therapy), this should be discussed during your sessions. Even if you don't tell him, your therapist should be able to discern your feelings of discomfort during the course of a session. In addition to your actual words, or lack of them, your nonverbal language should help clue him in to the fact that something is holding you back or upsetting you. Your therapist really has to work at being in tune with you—that's his job. If for some reason he hasn't perceived that something is troubling you, you should make every effort to tell him what is going on inside. A good therapist will have an arsenal of skills to help address these issues.

For example, if your therapist finds that you have uncomfortable feelings about therapy—or about him—he might make use of important techniques, such as *immediacy* and *self-disclosure*. Immediacy (also known as *you-me talk*) is the experience of and discussion about therapy itself, as well as the relationship between the therapist and the patient. This very direct approach brings the relationship you have with your therapist into view. Saying, "I sense that something is not right between us. Is there something going on between you and me that we should talk about?" is you-me talk. He might also say, "Did I miss something important that I should be focusing on?" Or, "You seem upset with me. Can we talk about that?" These are all examples of the use of immediacy by a therapist.

Additionally, your therapist might bring your nonverbal behavior into the open—into immediacy—by describing what he sees. "Since you came in you've been looking at the floor, and you haven't been as communicative as in the past. Also, your eyes seem a bit teary. I'm wondering if you are okay, and if you would like to tell me what you're thinking about." This kind of you-me talk helps the patient understand that the therapist is aware of, and cares about, him and the relationship.

Occasionally your therapist will use another technique, called *self-disclosure*, which is generally rarely used. Self-disclosure is a clinical technique that involves the telling of specific, limited amounts of personal information by a therapist. He might (briefly) tell you something about his own life that could inspire you and help you expand your understanding of your own issues. However, and this is a very big however, therapy should *never* be about your therapist. If he does use this technique, it should be used very sparingly, and it should be tailored to spur you to self-exploration. Also, he should never reveal intimate details about his relationships or use names.

Often, in order to steer the session toward inward exploration, your therapist will ask the kinds of open-ended questions that refer to your inner thoughts and feelings. They might come at the start of or during the session. "What were you thinking about right before your session, today?" or "What are you feeling right now?"

These questions are a bit more pointed than the open-ended ones we mentioned in the beginning of this chapter. As you become more and more comfortable with therapy, your therapist will use these questions in order to help you articulate feelings and thoughts you may not even know you have. He may even make this a part of the written treatment plan. After exploring your inner session further, you both may eventually decide to modify your treatment goals. Sometimes on a journey, if you catch a glimpse of a mountain or a valley, you'll want to examine the map and take a detour that will bring you to these yearned-for places. A skilled therapist knows when that detour is called for.

For example, if your primary treatment goal is to explore your fear of intimate relationships, but you arrive at each session feeling more and more depressed, after talking about your feelings, you and your therapist may come to the conclusion that your treatment goal should be redefined temporarily. Perhaps understanding and managing symptoms of depression would be a worthwhile goal. Conversely, there will be times when your therapist will want to help you focus on other important goals you may not even be aware of and may steer you gently toward them. Of course, he must have clinical justification for suggesting you focus on any specific problem. Ultimately, the feelings, emotions, thoughts, and behaviors you have during or in between sessions will all have a part to play in how therapy will unfold.

Until Next Time

No matter what happens during a session, whether or not you resolve an issue, as the end of the session approaches, your therapist should "check in" with you and make sure you are feeling okay. He may ask you to summarize your session by talking about your progress, discussing the accomplishments you made during the session, or exploring what you have achieved over the course of therapy so far. He may also summarize the session himself. He may also give you homework, highlighting some skills that you can work on before your next session. I like to give my patients a lot of homework—I want them to have really solid techniques at their fingertips to help them deal with both internal and external problems.

It is important that each session end on a positive, hopeful note. Above all, your therapist shouldn't allow the session to end if you are experiencing any extremely negative feelings or thoughts that might cause you to have a crisis. If you are overwhelmingly upset, he should encourage you to get a crisis evaluation, even if it means calling 911 for assistance. If he has another patient waiting to see him while you are experiencing a crisis, he should step out into the waiting room and ask the other patient if he would mind waiting or rescheduling. If when you leave you are still upset (though hopefully your feelings will be manageable), your therapist should ask you to call him later or offer to call you. I want to stress that ending a therapy session when you are in distress *should* be the rare exception rather than the rule.

Pay attention to this red flag: Unfortunately, there are therapists who are working out their own problems during their patients' therapy sessions. Some feel that they must "control" their patients. One of the easiest, most passive ways to do this is for them to allow a sensitive, vulnerable patient to leave while still upset. These therapists believe that a conflicted patient is more likely to return to therapy and keep coming back for an extended time in order to try and get rid of his bad feelings. Sometimes these therapists, either consciously or subconsciously, actually trigger the patient's bad feelings to keep him dependant and coming back for more therapy! Since these kinds of therapists obviously aren't the kinds of therapists who would teach their patients how to handle triggers in the first place, their patients are very vulnerable to this kind of manipulation.

If occasional strong, uncomfortable feelings appear to be the natural result of painful topics broached during your session, then you could be digging deep and doing the difficult work you may need to do. Effective therapy can cause feelings of discomfort. Experiencing feelings of sadness or anger during therapy is not unusual. However, if these bad feelings become habitual, or very extreme, then there is a problem. Pay attention: If these feelings seem to occur immediately before, during, or immediately after therapy, and occur *week after week*, then your clinical course of treatment may not be right for you. Speak to your therapist. Tell him what is going on. He should offer you solid solutions to this serious problem. If he doesn't, seek therapy elsewhere.

If your negative feelings just don't seem to go away at all or worsen over the period of a few months, then take a step back and process this with your therapist. Ask your therapist to review your treatment plan in some detail. Perhaps there are changes that need to be made. Perhaps you could consider medication or inpatient rehabilitation. Again, your therapist should explore the issue and then offer concrete solutions for you to try. If none of them work, an ethical therapist will recommend other courses of treatment or even another therapist. It is okay for you to take the lead and tell your therapist what you would like to focus on, or what course of action you think may be helpful. You have a right to be involved in determining your treatment (but not necessarily dictating it). For example, you may consider asking your therapist if he can recommend a psychiatrist who could prescribe a mild antidepressant or antianxiety medication that could be of help.

If your therapist doesn't address your negative feelings and help you explore and manage them, then he is not doing his job. The more clearly you can explain what is going on inside, and the more openly you can share this with your therapist, the more he will be able to help you and the more you will be able to help yourself. Sometimes keeping a journal while in therapy will help you in this area; additionally, a journal can help you assess whether or not this therapist is right for you. Other tools can also help you reflect on your situation.

The Personal Perspective Paper

A tool I created and often use to help patients record their problems (and successes) as they understand them is the *personal perspective paper* (PPP). The personal perspective paper is a useful therapeutic tool. It is a statement written or tape-recorded by the patient that describes his view of his problems and how they affect his life, his view of his progress, and how therapy is or isn't helping him. The PPP can be used at the beginning of therapy, at the end of therapy, and along the way, in some cases in order to help the patient reflect on his progress (or lack thereof) and help the therapist gain an "inside peek" at the patient's perspective.

When I ask patients to begin writing or tape-recording their *own* viewpoints on their problems, for many it is the first time they have faced their problems head-on, rather than sidling up and taking quick peeks at them. The most important perspective recorded in the initial PPP is how *you* think *your* problems are affecting *your* life. For example, someone who abuses prescription drugs may not really pay attention to exactly what this situation is doing to his life. When he works on his PPP, he will become very aware that these drugs are causing him to "check out" and not deal with problems at home or work. Or someone who has episodic anxiety may be unable to travel for fear of losing control on a plane or train. He may never have explored what this is doing to his personal and professional life. As he writes his PPP, he begins to see that he avoids many opportunities in life because of his fears. Exploring the impact of problems in all areas of life will help motivate you to change.

Also, the PPP is a valuable tool for measuring your clinical progress during the course of therapy. By writing down or otherwise recording your newly developing perspectives on your problems, you slow down and bring your life into focus. When you slow down and take time to articulate your feelings about the changes taking place, you get more in touch with yourself—you become more aware. At the end of therapy, too, another PPP can be written and compared to the initial PPP, affirming that, indeed, positive change has occurred.

The PPP will also help your therapist; it gives him another tool with which to understand you. If you have a severe problem, but in your initial PPP you minimize it (or vice versa), he will get insight into how you see yourself. If your perceptions of your progress (or lack of it) are radically different from his, he and you will be alerted to this by the PPP, and you will be able to process this. The initial PPP gives me an edge on understanding where my patients are coming from. I consider it optional, but useful.

Therapy Journal

Another helpful tool—one that many therapists recommend to their patients—is the therapy journal. For some, writing in a journal can help them zoom in on and clarify issues discussed during therapy. The entries in a therapy journal generally are about feelings, emotions, and thoughts; they may be about behaviors, too. By writing in a therapy journal before and after each session, the patient will be able to reflect in a more focused manner on the issues he is facing. Unlike the PPP, a journal is written in often, as much as several times a day.

Oddly enough, despite the intense focus on self, writing in a therapy journal can actually help you become less self-centered. By putting your deepest feelings and thoughts down on paper, you may leave room in your psyche to relate to the feelings and thoughts of others, and that will help you develop better relationships.

I believe, however, that there is another important role a therapy journal can play. It can be a detailed record of your sessions. Your entries can help you assess how therapy, or a particular therapist, is working for you. Talk about it with your therapist—a therapy journal may assist you in reaching your treatment goals.

Chapter 7

EXPERIENCED, ETHICAL, COMPETENT, AND CARING— OR NOT

I wonder men dare trust themselves with men.

—WILLIAM SHAKESPEARE, TIMON OF ATHENS

By now you will sense that the best relationships between therapist and patient are not just about clinical expertise. The bottom line is: they are also about trust. When your experienced, ethical, and competent therapist cares about you, trust blossoms. When you trust your therapist, you'll be able to confide in him, taking emotional risks that will help you reach your goals quickly and lastingly.

The therapist-patient relationship may be compared to the teacher-student relationship; just as the best teacher gives, expecting nothing in return but the growth of the student, the best therapist gives, expecting nothing in return but the healing of the patient. Like the teacher, the most successful therapist has one thing in abundance in addition to his professional skills: *empathy*. Empathy is the deep understanding of (and caring about) another's thoughts, feelings, and life situation. Although an ineffective therapist may or may not have empathy for his patients, a good therapist always does. He really cares.

Empathy: The Mirror and the Verbal Hug

After you have chosen your therapist and have worked with him for a few weeks, you should get the sense that he sincerely cares about your well-being. He may demonstrate this overtly by actively listening to you. He also will regularly repeat back to you what you tell him, simply, in his own words. He will condense, clarify, and sum up what you say. If you tell him, for example, "I keep oversleeping and missing job interviews. I can't seem to go to sleep at night or get up in the morning. I am feeling really bad about this; I'm crying all the time, and eating too much chocolate," your therapist could say something like, "It seems like you are unhappy with your inability to move forward and make the most of opportunities. You are having problems getting to sleep at night, and this makes it hard to keep important appointments. This seems to be making you feel really bad and is fueling your desire to overeat chocolate." By paraphrasing what you say in therapy, your therapist is showing you that he has really heard you and understands what you are saying. He is also acting like a reflection in a mirror. When you hear what you are saying repeated back to you, you will be able to step back and find new ways of understanding what is going on. Mirroring is a way to help you reframe experiences.

Another way your therapist can show you he has empathy for you is by reaching out to you, genuinely sympathizing with your pain, and when you are ready, helping you let go of pain. By verbally sharing his concern for you, he is giving you a verbal hug. This will reassure you that your therapist really does care. Remember, though, the "hug" should be verbal and should never make you feel violated in any way. Respecting your boundaries and keeping the demarcation between therapist and patient very firm is extremely important.

In the following true therapy tales, some of which are very upsetting, boundaries were broken and empathy was in short supply. Because there are so many ethical, caring, and dedicated therapists out there, we want to emphasize that these experiences are not representative of most therapy experiences. However, by reading about bad therapy practices, we believe you'll be better prepared to know what to avoid and to seek the kind of care you deserve. In order to make very clear what are suspect practices, beneath each story in this chapter are red flag violations—basic rules of therapy that were violated by the therapist. You'll also note that these red flags almost never occur singly. That's because even though no therapist, and indeed no person, is perfectly professional at all times, if a therapist is willing to violate even one of these basic rules, he probably is willing to violate more.

Sleight of Mind

Madeline is bright and sophisticated, successful in her career as a museum curator and a loyal and well-loved daughter, sister, and friend. Still, like many of us, she was searching for more meaning in her life. She also had lingering anxieties and fears after the death of her brother that she wanted to deal with. She decided that perhaps therapy could help her. A colleague at work recommended Dr. Phelps, a psychotherapist in Madeline's Florida town—by all accounts reputable and experienced—who unfortunately, as Madeline was soon to learn, charged far more than her services were worth. Dr. Phelps's fee for an office visit was $250 per hour, and she had no qualms about doing therapy sessions on the phone at the same rate. In addition to a great willingness to do therapy sessions over the phone, there were other red flags.

Dr. Phelps was chronically late for sessions, sometimes by as much as thirty minutes. She did apologize for her tardiness, but Madeline felt frustrated because this happened session after session. Also, Dr. Phelps suggested to Madeline that her lateness was a legitimate therapeutic technique that she was using in order to more effectively treat Madeline. This excuse—and abuse—masquerading as therapy was a very creative and manipulative "sleight of mind." Dr. Phelps pretended that her behavior was a type of "confrontational therapy." She actually made these excuses up in order to draw Madeline's attention away from her egregious unprofessional behavior and cover up her clear lack of empathy. She would rather hurt her patient than correct her own failings.

Madeline (naturally) felt that Dr. Phelps was "goading" her into anger. It gave Madeline the very justifiable impression that Dr. Phelps was "fraudulent and disrespectful." She offered Madeline no clinical justification for the "techniques" she was using, and Madeline sensed that something was way off base. Still, it took several months before Madeline could extricate herself from Dr. Phelps's web of deceit. Any patient, no matter how intelligent, is in a vulnerable position, and instead of building genuine trust, Dr. Phelps took advantage of Madeline's vulnerability.

She gave many other indications that she did not genuinely care about Madeline. During the $250-per-hour phone sessions that took place (again, phone sessions are not something I recommend unless there is an emergency), Madeline would hear Dr. Phelps caring for her dog. Clearly, she wasn't caring for Madeline.

When after eight months Madeline finally had the courage to ask Dr. Phelps when she could expect to see progress in her treatment, Dr. Phelps accused of her of not trusting her and implied that something was wrong with Madeline for having the temerity to ask. Needless to say, Madeline never saw a treatment plan, so she had no way of getting a clear picture of what the goals of her therapy were. She had no real understanding that it was Dr. Phelps's job to work together with her to bring about positive change. Dr. Phelps also never gave Madeline a treatment time line, so therapy would have continued to drag on indefinitely if Madeline hadn't finally realized that it was going nowhere.

Despite conflicted feelings, Madeline decided to leave. She still had much guilt and confusion for more than a year after she made her decision. Now, though much time has passed, one can sense the bewilderment and pain this experience caused Madeline. She lost faith in the therapy process. Fortunately for her, she has moved on. Unfortunately for others, Dr. Phelps is still running a busy practice.

Red Flag Violations:

1. **Chronic Tardiness:** If a therapist cannot respect your time, he cannot respect you.
2. **Manipulation and Dishonesty:** If a therapist tries to cover up failings or errors, especially if he says his failings or errors are actually "part of your therapy," this shows that he lacks foundational morals.

3. **Emotional Blackmail/Control:** If a therapist tells you that if you don't blindly trust him, he feels hurt and/or something is wrong with you, he is trying to use emotional appeals to control you. *Emotional blackmail* involves several forms of manipulation that can be subtly passive-aggressive or overtly aggressive. By the use of emotional blackmail, a person aims to control another and/or force another to do what the perpetrator wants by subtly or overtly threatening consequences, such as inducing overwhelming guilt in the victim.

4. **Regular Phone Sessions:** The phone is okay to use for occasional emergency sessions or as an adjunct to in-person sessions in times of crisis or stress, but not as a replacement for in-person sessions (some therapists disagree).

5. **Lack of Respect for Session Time:** Caring for dogs during sessions, answering nonemergency phone calls, or doing anything that takes a therapist's attention away from you shows a profound disrespect for you, your time, and the fee you are paying him.

6. **Lack of Therapy Basics:** If you have no treatment plan, no treatment goals, and no time frame in which to work on those goals, how are you and your therapist going to know when you are done with therapy?

7. **Lack of Empathy:** If a therapist seems to display a lack of caring about your feelings, talk about it with him right away! If unempathetic behavior continues, this is your cue—this person should not be in a profession where caring about others is a basic personality requirement. Move on!

Blurring Boundaries and Borders

Lisa was a very "together" person. She graduated from an Ivy League school with honors. Although she excelled in math, her greatest talents lay in her ability to use words well. She was able to explain difficult concepts in terms anyone could understand. This helped her get a job at a prestigious company that developed math textbooks. Her sizzling (and wry) sense of humor made her extremely popular both at work and in her social life—she had many friends and acquaintances. Lisa was always able to make them laugh. She was also in a stable, loving, long-term relationship and had close relationships with her parents and siblings.

During her early thirties, Lisa began to feel unable to cope with an abusive relative, a cousin with whom she owned a house inherited from her grandfather. Without her knowledge, he managed to seize control of the property. It was a very painful blow to Lisa, especially because she saw him frequently. In her prestigious Los Angeles neighborhood, there were few psychologists as respected as Dr. Dallas Grasse, so that is who she turned to when she decided to get help.

Though we won't focus here on many of the red flags of Lisa's therapy experience, we want to mention some in brief. Dr. Grasse didn't write a treatment plan. She kept Lisa in therapy for more than five years, though she had no signs of any serious mental illness, and, indeed, just came to therapy to work on managing her anger at her cousin. But Dallas did appear to be empathetic and concerned about Lisa's well-being. Lisa liked Dallas from day one. She looked forward to her therapy sessions. Even though she didn't have a treatment plan or goals, she felt she was getting something from therapy— she noticed that she was far less angry with her cousin than when she started.

However, all that started to change when Dallas began to share with Lisa the details of a special program for hospitals she and her psychology consulting company were in the process of developing. The program was designed to help patients' families with the stresses of having a loved one in the hospital. It encouraged the use of psychotherapy as part of the healing process.

Lisa thought the program sounded great. She believed it would be fun to work with Dallas. She felt that it wouldn't be unethical for her to work for Dallas's program while she was still in therapy. She suggested the idea, and after "talking it through," Dallas agreed. She knew Lisa not only could write all her organization's literature, but could help her design a website as well. They agreed upon an hourly rate, and Lisa went to work.

Sometimes during therapy sessions the topic would naturally drift toward the work Lisa was doing for Dallas. But when it did, Dallas didn't charge her for these sessions, although she did use up her scheduled time on these occasions. Clearly, Dallas thought her own work was more pressing than Lisa's need for therapy. If that were the case, why did she still allow Lisa to keep scheduling appointments?

After Lisa completed the initial phase of the project (assisting in the building of the website, creating the text for promotional literature, and more), she received tons of praise, not only from Dallas, but from her coworkers as well. Then one Wednesday, several months after she started the project, she turned in the bill for her work. Two days later, on Friday, shortly after 5:00 PM, Lisa received an e-mail from Dallas. In impersonal language, it said that they could no longer afford Lisa's services and that she was being let go. Dallas signed off by saying she would see Lisa Monday, at her next therapy session.

At that session, Lisa confronted Dallas. She told her how unprofessional it was that she was fired in an e-mail. She said that any employer—not to mention one with whom she had a therapeutic relationship—would at least tell someone they were fired in person or on the phone. In response, Dallas went on the attack. "I see you still have your anger problem. I have failed you as a therapist." Lisa, though, did not take this manipulative statement lying down. She said, "How dare you say those things to me. You are sitting in judgment of me—that is your failure. You have violated what should be a safe environment. You could have really done me harm, but I am stronger than that." Dallas didn't respond and Lisa walked out, never to return.

Of course, by now you recognize some of the red flag violations that also appeared in Lisa's experience: lack of therapy basics, including a treatment plan and time frame for therapy; lack of empathy by firing Lisa, despite her being a patient (not to mention sheer, unmitigated chutzpah—firing Lisa *in an impersonal e-mail*). *Boundaries* or *borders* in therapy are the necessary dividing lines between individuals that maintain the healthy differences between people of different backgrounds, roles, status, sex, and individualities. The foundational violation in this case—the most confusing of all violations— was a blurring of boundaries.

Red Flag Violations:

1. **Blurring of boundaries:** When a therapist's and patient's lives intersect in some kind of relationship outside of therapy (except for occasional overlaps, such as the therapist shops at a store where the patient is a clerk), this is a no-no. A therapist who hires a patient he is currently treating is engaging in an egregious violation of therapy ethics. Having a professional or interpersonal relationship with a therapist is confusing, at best, and can possibly cause severe emotional suffering.

2. **Lacking Therapy Basics:** Can lead to . . .

3. **Endless Therapy:** When therapy goes on, and on, and on (except, of course, in cases of patients suffering from mental illness who may need long-term or even lifelong, therapy), there's something wrong. Endless therapy is a moneymaking maneuver, plain and simple.

4. **Lack of Empathy:** Firing anyone in an e-mail would be cruel, even if it wasn't your therapist (the person you pay to really care about your feelings) doing it.

5. **Manipulation:** If your therapist proclaims that he is a failure because you are angry at him or shows some other "off" emotion you find unpalatable, this is a dodge. And a weird one at that.

Hit-and-run and Hit-and-stay Therapy

Angelica had a tough time growing up. Her father walked out when she was eight and then her mother remarried two years later and gave up custody of her to her sister. Angelica was then raised by an aunt who viewed Angelica as a great burden and said so—constantly. When she turned eighteen, she was told to move out. She left her aunt's house in the suburbs, rented a room in the city, got a job as a waitress, took some college courses in psychology, and decided she would go to therapy. She had enough insight to know that she hadn't had the greatest familial role models, and she wanted to sort out her feelings so one day she would be able to marry and raise a family.

Carol, her boss at the restaurant where Angelica worked, recommended that she try Dr. Leslie Ellis, a psychologist who was very expensive, but who had helped her son with behavioral issues. She even gave Angelica a loan to help pay for some sessions. Angelica arrived at her first appointment with high hopes.

The building was in a very trendy neighborhood, and the office interior was clearly the work of a cutting-edge designer, but Leslie's wardrobe was conservative—tailored, elegant, and very expensive. She greeted Angelica when she arrived and showed her to a comfortable armchair, while she sat on a sleek leather sofa. Draped over the sofa was a plush fur coat that Leslie occasionally stroked during the session, with her beautifully manicured fingers, as if it were a kitten. Leslie began by asking Angelica why she came to see her. Angelica began to tell her story.

Leslie nodded and made sympathetic noises throughout the session, making Angelica feel very comfortable. She was really able to open up. Leslie didn't, however, talk about a treatment plan or help Angelica formulate manageable treatment goals, though Angelica herself asked about these things since she was studying psychology. "Shouldn't I have a treatment plan?" she asked the doctor. But Leslie said that the use of a treatment plan would "hamper her style" of therapy. Angelica said okay.

During the second session, right before the hour was up, Leslie suggested to Angelica that she was much "sicker" than she had thought originally. She told her that her request for a treatment plan might indicate a perverse need for control. She said that Angelica would have to come to therapy two or three times a week to "get to the bottom of her sickness."

Angelica was devastated. She told Carol what happened, told her she would not be able to afford to go back to college the next semester because she needed to use all her money for therapy, and asked for extra waitress shifts in order to pay for therapy. Carol, to her credit, said, "Something seems fishy." She told Angelica that although she knew she had a hard life, she was doing remarkably well, and that, in fact, she was one of the sanest people she knew. Carol told her that at her next session she should ask Leslie exactly how long all this therapy would take. Angelica agreed.

Shortly after the session began, Leslie asked her patient if she had given any more thought to increasing the frequency of her sessions. Angelica said she had, but that she had some questions first. She told Leslie that the cost of therapy was prohibitive; she was a college student who worked as a waitress to support herself—there was no other source of income. Leslie told Angelica that she would find a way to cut back on other expenses if her mental health was important to her. "For example," Leslie told her, "You mentioned you take the subway here. Why don't you walk? It's only twenty blocks or so."

Angelica told Leslie that she took the subway because she was always pressed for time, and that this brought her to her next concern after money, which was time.

"How many months of therapy will I need if I come to see you twice a week?"

Leslie thought for a moment. "Well, dear, you see, with your family history, you will most likely be in therapy for the rest of your life."

Angelica felt as if she had been hit by a hammer. She watched Leslie stroking her fur, as if in slow motion. She repeated the words "the rest of my life" out loud. Then she had a lightning flash of insight: "This woman is just trying to take my money and has no qualms about telling me I am sick in order to do so." She stood up, looked the very shocked therapist in the eye, and said, "I don't think so. In fact, I am not coming back to you again. I don't want my therapy to pay for your designer lifestyle."

Red Flag Violations:

1. **Lack of Empathy:** If a therapist is aware that a patient has extreme financial restrictions but is not willing to either work within the patient's existing budget or refer the patient to a therapist or clinic he or she can afford; if a therapist is also willing to hurt the patient in order to manipulate the patient's emotions (especially right before a session ends), this shows a serious lack of empathy.

2. **Lack of Therapy Basics and Refusal to Work with Them when Requested:** It's one thing for a therapist to "wing it" and not use a

treatment plan. We argue that it is unprofessional. It is, however, quite another thing to refuse to write a treatment plan when asked. I would argue that this shows an even more profound . . .

3. **Lack of Professionalism and Respect for a Patient:** Perhaps that's why a therapist like Leslie, in order to keep patients, had to resort to . . .

4. **Hit-and-stay Therapy:** When a therapist makes a pronouncement (often in the form of an extreme diagnosis), in order to keep a patient in endless therapy, this is what I call *hit-and-stay therapy*, a close relative of . . .

5. **Hit-and-run Therapy:** If a therapist makes a hurtful pronouncement about the state of your mental health, especially when this comes at the end of a session and you have no time to process what is said, this is what I call *hit-and-run therapy*. The therapist hurts the patient and leaves him hanging, unable to resolve the pain. This is designed to keep the patient "sick" and off-balance. It also leads the naive and vulnerable patient to believe that the only way to resolve his "sickness" is with . . .

6. **The Therapy Trap** aka **Endless Therapy:** Funded, of course, by the patient.

The Angry Therapist

Paris and Donovan were young, stylish, and newly wed. Donovan was a successful writer and Paris was a portrait painter. They both had strong family connections and shared similar values and goals, but like many newlyweds, found the first year or two of marriage to be stressful. In addition to dynamic careers, they had baby Oliver less than a year after the wedding. Life was busy!

When Oliver was still an infant, Paris and Donovan, being proactive go-getters, decided that perhaps they should seek out some counseling to help them navigate and negotiate the terms of their relationship. A friend told them about Dr. Lange, a respected psychologist in private practice not too far from their Philadelphia neighborhood. Dr. Lange, it turned out, was the head of a prestigious psychological association.

Paris and Donovan scheduled a session with Dr. Lange. He charged $200 for a fifty-minute session—a practice I am not fond of. I think most patients need a full hour of therapy, and the last ten minutes should be spent helping the patient wind up the session and prepare to leave. I believe the therapist should then, as a rule, schedule a ten- to fifteen-minute break in which to write his session notes. Yes, this may mean he won't be able to see as many patients in a day, but he will be able to focus more and do a better job. Cutting out ten minutes of the patient's face-to-face time in order to write notes seems like cheating to me, somehow.

Oliver and Paris decided to see Dr. Lange and went to three sessions together. At the end of the third session, he told them that Paris was the one in need of therapy because she had emotional problems, whereas Donovan had only practical problems he could solve by himself. Not knowing much about family counseling or individual therapy, they complied with his recommendation and Paris began to go to weekly individual therapy sessions without Donovan.

There was no treatment plan. No treatment goals were even discussed. The session followed the same pattern every week. Paris gave it her all—she was highly motivated, and so she talked and talked about her feelings, her relationships, her behavior, and more, all as honestly as she was able, but Dr. Lange gave her little or no direction or feedback. After several sessions, in which she saw little or no input from Dr. Lange, Paris decided she needed to understand more about the therapy process. "I asked him where therapy was going and what I could expect from it. He told me I had to 'wait and see,' and that I had to 'trust him,' and that the therapy process just 'happened.'" After several more sessions, Paris still felt like nothing was happening. Of course, she was most likely correct. She decided to ask Dr. Lange again for more feedback, this time a bit more assertively.

"I asked him to explain the therapy process to me. I described to him what I do for a living. I told him that although I couldn't actually teach someone to paint a portrait in the space of a brief conversation, I could explain the basic process; how I prepared the sitter, the setting, and the lighting; the tools I needed, like paints and brushes and canvas; and about how long it would take. I told him, 'I'm hoping that you can give me the same kind of overview of therapy so I can understand what is going on in these sessions.'"

Dr. Lange appeared to be stunned by her question. "He said, 'Incredible! What? You want me to tell you here in this office, in the next half hour what I learned in four years of psychological studies?'" Before he was finished, Paris felt so bad for offending him that she spent the rest of the session apologizing to him. She experienced very mixed feelings and felt off balance. At a subsequent session, after she tentatively questioned him again, Dr. Lange told her she simply must trust him. "How can you expect to ever trust your husband if you don't trust me"?

Paris was upset. She let the subject go for several sessions, but still felt very off balance (as well she should—Dr. Lange was manipulating her and taking advantage of her vulnerability). "I had made myself very open, but somehow I felt that my failure to get anything out of therapy was my fault, so I kept on putting myself emotionally into it. Also, another weird thing about this was that Dr. Lange kept implying that part of my therapy was the actual act of me being kept in suspense. He even told me that I needed to understand that it was good for me to 'not have too much information.'"

After a few more months of sessions, she decided to try once more to speak directly to the doctor. "'I put myself on the line, but nothing much seems to be happening,' I told him. 'How long is therapy going to take?'"

"'Don't worry,' he told me, 'I won't keep you for a long time. You just have to let therapy work.'" But Paris didn't take this vague reply at face value this time. She repeated her questions.

Dr. Lange's demeanor changed dramatically. "If you weren't going to trust my expertise, you shouldn't have come to see *me* in the first place. You should have done your research and chosen another therapist," he said snidely. After this outburst, Paris finally decided that she and her husband needed to discuss this turn of events.

Donovan did not want to give up on Dr. Lange yet. He thought that maybe this is what therapy is like. Who were they to know how therapy worked? Perhaps they should still give him the benefit of the doubt? They decided that they should try to talk to Dr. Lange together. Paris called him. "I told him that I don't understand the therapeutic process. I asked him if maybe he could talk to my husband, explain it to him, and then he could clarify things for me. Dr. Lange was very cold when I asked him this and refused to see us together in person, but he grudgingly agreed that we could schedule a three-way phone call."

Paris asked Donovan to take charge, and he did. "When we called Dr. Lange, he immediately sounded defensive. Donovan asked him to help them understand where therapy was going, and he responded in an exasperated tone of voice, 'I *told* her so many times already.'"

"He was so over-the-top emotional, even acrimonious. I was on another extension. Donovan and I looked over at each other in surprise."

The therapist began what can only be described as a rant. "In all my years of therapy, I have never had a spouse call and interfere like this. Frankly, your calling is messing up the entire course of therapy. You are controlling your wife and you are overly possessive. You are afraid therapy is going to work, and then Paris won't be under your control anymore. And you, Paris, are manipulating Donovan."

During our conversation, Paris explained, "It was unbelievable. He clearly hated us, even me, his patient."

Needless to say, the couple never went back. There were so many examples of unprofessional, unacceptable behavior on the part of Dr. Lange that long after the incident, the confusion and pain in Paris's voice as she tells the story is palpable. If your therapist refuses to take your questions about therapy seriously enough to answer in a direct, clear manner that you are able to understand, run—don't walk—to the nearest exit.

Red Flag Violations:

1. **Manipulation and Dishonesty:** If a therapist suggests to a patient that not having vital information (needed by the patient in order to help him understand and feel comfortable with therapy) is "part of

the therapy," then the therapist is trying to control the patient, quite dishonestly. Paris's experience with this was similar to Madeline's experience with her therapist telling her that her chronic lateness was a part of her "therapy."

2. **Emotional Blackmail and Control:** Telling a patient that she should have chosen another therapist and that she should just be able to trust him is designed to unsettle and control her. It is, frankly, playing unfair. It could also go under the heading of manipulation and dishonesty. "How can you expect to ever trust your husband if you don't trust me?" is evidence of controlling the patient by posing an unanswerable, attacking question.

3. **Lack of Respect for Patient (and Husband):** If a therapist refuses to answer questions directly or name calls, as Dr. Lange did during the phone call with Donovan and Paris, or if he manipulates, bullies, emotionally blackmails, and tries to control a patient, that is all evidence of a profound lack of respect as well as a . . .

4. **Lack of Empathy:** He doesn't care if you suffer and doesn't care if he's the cause of your suffering.

5. **Lack of Therapy Basics:** No treatment plan, no treatment goals, and an unwillingness to discuss these things, and implying that wanting to know where therapy is headed is actually a failing of the patient, all adds up to . . .

6. **Lack of Professionalism (Arrogance and Anger):** Displays of anger and intolerance upon being questioned, an inability to not take things personally, viewing questions or concerns as being about himself, and displaying hubris all speak of a therapist who is not, first and foremost, professional, and second, not emotionally mature enough to be a therapist. The greatest indication of this is that he . . .

7. **Blames the Patient.**

Sleepy Doc

No, that's not the name of two of the seven dwarfs, but what we call a therapist who is far less interested in you than he should be. José was a rather high-energy, late-night, party-loving guy who was finding he had bouts of unmanageable anxiety. So, when he met his new therapist, Larry, an experienced social worker, he noticed what seemed like a big plus right away—Larry was very calm, even laid-back. Larry also accepted José's insurance plan.

After discussing Larry with his wife, Marie (who hoped that Larry's calming influence would scale back her husband's sometimes off-the-wall, late-night antics, which seemed to trigger his anxiety), José agreed to try working with Larry. Larry did many things right. He wrote a treatment plan with José. He was also punctual and seemed like a very warm person, at least initially. The first three sessions that took place in the afternoons went very well. But then José's work schedule changed. He asked Larry to meet at night, preferably after 9:00, and Larry agreed. But four sessions later José began to feel that he just couldn't connect to Larry anymore. He felt that therapy was not going to work.

Marie was a social worker and had worked with me a few years before this situation developed. She called me to ask if José could briefly talk with me. He was having some questions about Larry. I said sure. José and Marie were living in Colorado at the time and I was in New York, so I didn't even know who Larry was. I could give a fairly unbiased opinion.

José's description of his therapy sessions sounded a bit "off." It seemed like José did virtually all the talking and was getting very little response, which is not how his therapy started out. I asked José what Larry's face looked like as he listened to José talk. José said, "I have no idea. He sits at an angle to my chair, and the light from a floor lamp reflects off his glasses."

I told José to move his chair, and be sure he could look directly into Larry's eyes. Well, we both got a big surprise. At the next session José did as I suggested. It seemed that most of the time the psychotherapist's eyes were closed. In fact, it looked like once or twice he was even nodding off. It turned out that Larry was dozing during José's appointments!

José wasn't shy. He waited until Larry had fallen asleep (which happened about fifteen minutes into his next session), then shook his arm lightly to wake him. He then told Larry that he had fallen asleep and that this had been going on for a while. Larry, to his credit, apologized sincerely, and told José that he was just exhausted by the time José showed up for his evening appointments. He said he hadn't been quite sure he was falling asleep and was embarrassed. He offered to see José for four free sessions to make up for the sessions during which he had fallen asleep.

Because Larry was honest and really seemed to care, and had also agreed to not charge for the sessions during which he slept, José decided to give it another try. He was glad he did. Larry really helped him learn how to calm down, taught him relaxation exercises, and encouraged him to work off his stress by playing basketball. I guess Larry's ability to doze off during sessions showed that he was just the right kind of person to teach relaxation techniques. He also worked with José on other issues that came up. It was a fruitful therapy relationship.

Red Flag Violation:

Not Responsive/Not Using Session Time Wisely: Letting a patient talk without responding—especially falling asleep—is not okay! This was an unusual case, one where the therapist was truly experienced, ethical, competent, and, as it turns out, caring. However, if a therapist regularly seems bored, sleepy, or uninterested in you during your session time, this is certainly a topic to be explored further. Remember: Your therapist is paid to be interested in you. It is not your job to entertain him or keep him awake.

Thrifty Ways to Leave Your Therapist

If you spot minor red flag violations during therapy, talk about them with your therapist. If his response is not defensive and he is willing to take what you say seriously and correct any deficiencies, then you should continue working with him. Sometimes a simple misunderstanding could be perceived by a patient as a flagrant violation. Sometimes a violation really did occur. The chances of these violations happening to you will be greatly reduced because you will have followed the interview and reference-checking process in this book. There are many terrific therapists, both in clinics and in private practice, who are experienced, ethical, competent, and caring—you just have to put the effort into finding the right one.

But let's suppose for a moment that you have been working with a therapist who has sent up a few red flags. When you politely question him, he gets defensive and blames you for any problems in therapy. Maybe he refuses, in his most warm and winning manner, to write a treatment plan when asked. Or perhaps you have been in therapy with someone for months, or even years, and you feel you are reading about him as you read this chapter. Wow. Is that *my* therapist who is so unethical? You realize it is time to leave your therapist—at this point asking your therapist to write a treatment plan, discuss a time frame for therapy, discuss treatment goals, stop manipulating you, and so on will not be productive.

It's important to understand two main things before you decide how to let a therapist know you will not be continuing with him: (1) where you are, emotionally speaking, and (2) the nature of your grievances. So how do you do it? How do you leave a bad therapist? Here are some possibilities; there may be more.

Ending Therapy over the Phone

If you are annoyed and angry that you have wasted time and money with a therapist and don't want to pay for anymore sessions, then don't schedule another session in which to fire your therapist—why should you pay him more money? Just call him on the phone and tell him that you won't need his services anymore. You can tell him that you are moving forward, or that you no longer have time or room in your budget for therapy. I don't recommend you discuss why you are letting him go if his neglect has been serious; if he is someone who is unethical and manipulative, the conversation could be very uncomfortable for you. He could also try to talk you into scheduling just "one more appointment." That isn't necessary if he is a flagrant red flag violator.

If you are feeling very vulnerable, still in need of therapy, but know that this therapist is not for you, call and cancel your next appointment and say that at present you are not ready to schedule another appointment. This will give you time to find another therapist. You can tell your new therapist what happened and sign a release giving him permission to speak to your old therapist. He can call or write to him, requesting session notes and treatment plans (if any have been made) so that there is some basic continuity of treatment. This way your old therapist will certainly get the message that his services are no longer required.

If your therapist has caused you to feel very threatened, or you feel you simply cannot cope with speaking to him again or even writing him, try calling his voice mail when you know he won't pick up and leave a message saying you will no longer be coming to appointments. Or if you feel you have no other option, just don't show up. I hesitate to recommend this—it is really a last resort and should only be used if a therapist has been extremely negligent and abusive.

Dear Sigmund Letter: A Sample Farewell Letter

If you feel you would like to tell your therapist the reasons why you are leaving, and get them off your chest, go right ahead—but do it on paper or via e-mail. And if possible, have a wise friend or other advisor take a look at what you wrote. Make sure it is honest, even passionate and emotional, if you feel that being emotional will help you move on, but it shouldn't be abusive. Don't threaten the therapist, don't use inappropriate language, and don't call names. Here's an example of what you might write.

Dear Sigmund,

I am writing this letter to tell you why I will no longer continue to use your services as a therapist. I entered therapy with high hopes—my problems weren't serious, but I wanted to improve myself and my relationships with others. I was also feeling blue and worried that I might be depressed. I was prepared to work hard and do what it took to fulfill my highest potential. I kept my part of the bargain. I paid you promptly for each session, I almost always showed up on time, and I followed whatever recommendations you made. I relied on you to help me improve my life.

But you didn't keep up your part of the bargain. You didn't take a comprehensive biopsychosocial history. You didn't develop a treatment plan for me, and when I asked you to, you said you had the treatment plan in your "head." You rarely took notes during sessions or afterward. I know because your next patient always came in as I was walking out the door. You were occasionally late for appointments but never offered an apology, as I did the one time I was late.

You did listen to me, but I was paying you for more than listening—I was paying you to help me define and reach personal goals. Though unvoiced, my goals do exist. They were just hidden beneath the surface, waiting for you to help me draw them out. I aim to live a better life for myself, my family, and for everyone I interact with. That is why I am moving on to work with a therapist who will work with me on a plan to help me accomplish this. To the best of my understanding, that is what my therapy with you should have been about but wasn't.

I believe that you probably want to be a good therapist. I can't pretend to know why you didn't give me the foundational services essential to quality treatment. I hope that you take my criticism in the spirit it was intended— and that you improve so that your current patients and future patients really benefit from seeing you instead of wasting their time and money.

Sincerely,

Your former patient

Although you may be in the position where you have to choose one of these options, I hope you're not. I have worked with hundreds of psychotherapists over the years, and most of them have been deeply concerned about their patients and have worked very hard to become good therapists. I hope that this is the kind of therapist you are seeing.

Chapter 8

WHAT'S HOLDING ME BACK?

The only use of an obstacle is to be overcome.

—WOODROW WILSON

It seems that a large percentage of patients that my colleagues and I treat have previously been in therapy with at least one, and usually more than one, therapist. Perhaps the most pervasive form of bad therapy practices that patients engage in is the *therapy-go-round*, a situation in which an individual goes from therapist to therapist and continuously receives ineffectual treatment in a seemingly never-ending search for an effective treatment for his problems. Why is this the case? I don't have definitive answers, but based on many years of discussions with therapists and patients, I believe that there are several contributing factors.

Financial Concerns

Not necessarily the leading factor, but certainly a common one, is concern about money. When a patient can't afford to continue a course of (effective) therapy, and he stops before his treatment goals are fully reached, he will usually find it difficult to maintain momentum and complete his treatment goals on his own. He will often stagnate or backslide. Because the therapy he did get was effective and he saw that it helped him, the next time he has funds available, he may try therapy again. Of course, his insurance or cash funds can run out again and again. When a patient stops and starts courses of therapy, it drains his spirit and his pocketbook. After an overabundance of aborted attempts, he is broke, both financially and emotionally. His problems still exist.

Another common way money can be a factor that leads to a ride on the therapy-go-round is when a patient uses his therapy budget (whether insurance allotments or cash funds) to complete an *ineffective* course of treatment. He still feels as bad (or worse) as when he started therapy. He is now back where he started, only with less money in his pocket. He may have to wait to seek more (and hopefully, better) therapy and lives in a kind of limbo until he is able to do so.

I strongly urge you to explore low-cost therapy options if either of the above two scenarios seems to describe your situation. There are many excellent therapists who work on a *sliding scale*, or a fee based on a patient's ability to pay (therefore a patient with a higher income would pay a higher fee than a patient with a lower income), as well as those who work in low-cost, free, or nearly free community or government-funded clinics (find out about the latter on your state government's website). Many qualified therapists work part- or full-time in state-funded or other clinics while also maintaining their own private practices; don't hesitate to ask a therapist in private practice if he does so. Some even do pro bono work privately or for not-for-profit clinics. As mentioned before, though some superb therapists charge a very high fee, many don't. An expensive therapist is not necessarily a good therapist.

Feeling Disconnected

The next factor that may cause people to go round and round with one therapist after another is a "connection" problem. Most patients are able to connect with quality therapists because the therapists create an atmosphere that supports engagement. However, when patients aren't satisfied because they feel their needs aren't being addressed by their therapists, they leave and seek another therapist or give up on therapy altogether.

Sometimes patients let therapy drag on until they find a new therapist or they let the feelings of dissatisfaction build up until they reach the point of total frustration and then suddenly quit. Either right away or after a time, they search for someone new. I urge all those who are dissatisfied with a therapist to confront him. Tell him why you aren't happy with therapy. Your reasons may very well be valid. Give your therapist the chance to correct any methods or other issues that are alienating you. Remember, you can be your own best advocate. (Note: In situations where your therapist is abusive, do not confront a therapist—find a new therapist as quickly as possible.)

One of the best ways to thwart connection problems is by using a treatment plan (see Chapter 5). Ideally, at the start of therapy your needs (which can be implicit in your objectives and goals) will be addressed and written into the treatment plan. Then you and your therapist will be able to work in unison toward common, agreed-upon goals. If you have a comprehensive treatment plan set up, you will find out very early on if a particular course of therapy and/or therapist is potentially effective. Remember: if a need has been overlooked and has not been made a part of the treatment plan, or an unexpected need has arisen during the course of therapy, it can be addressed at any point.

It is in some measure up to you to describe your needs to your therapist. Yes, your therapist should be in tune with you and ask you probing questions that help him to understand what you need, but at the same time, he isn't a psychic. Help him to help you; tell him if you feel something is lacking in the therapy process and tell him you want to address it—together.

Therapist Hopping

Sometimes people hop from one qualified, even excellent, therapist to another. They seek that elusive someone who will make their world a better place and fulfill their needs and desires. Some are looking for a high, a feeling of self-validation, not unlike people who go from bar to bar looking to have an intense new experience or to meet the person who will give their life meaning. Alcohol, music, and sometimes drugs augment the barhopper's futile search; these things, as well as emotional highs, can augment the patient's search as well.

The personality factors that lead to this type of therapist hopping can be insidious—and very painful for a patient to confront in himself. The presence of personality disorders wreak havoc on an individual's life and could lead him (or others associated with him) to seek therapy. *Personality disorders* are several varied types of mental disorders in which the individual has rigid (and often self-destructive) patterns of thought and behavior that remain the same no matter what the situation. Those with personality disorders do not think or act appropriately and are usually difficult to treat. There are ten specific types (and a catchall unspecified type) of these disorders, but most are generally characterized by at least some of the following: frequent mood swings, angry outbursts and rage, distrust of others, serious problems making friends and sustaining relationships, lack of empathy, poor impulse control, and alcohol or substance abuse.

Many of the ten specific personality disorders are considered extremely difficult to treat. Some of these include:

- **Borderline Personality Disorder:** predominant elements of which feature a pattern of unstable relationships, confused self-image, and extremely impulsive behavior.
- **Narcissistic Personality Disorder:** predominant elements of which are a pattern of grandiosity, extreme need for admiration, and lack of empathy.
- **Histrionic Personality Disorder:** predominant elements of which are extreme attention seeking and a pattern of displaying excessively emotional behavior.

These and other difficult-to-treat personality disorders may be a factor in why some patients skip from therapist to therapist. For example, patients with histrionic personality disorder want to feel special, more fascinating, and more loved than other people. They may expect praise or even worship from others. Anyone who doesn't give that praise, including a therapist, may be treated to a hysterical tantrum. If the therapist doesn't appease the patient, he may be struck off the list of acceptable companions.

The patient with histrionic personality disorder can often feel hollow and empty and seeks therapy in order to help with those feelings. However, those who do seek treatment often therapist hop until they find the therapist able to satisfy their endless need for attention. In addition to demanding admiration, these patients may try to manipulate and control others with overly emotional behavior, changing lists of symptoms, and even by giving extravagant or inappropriate gifts.

An experienced therapist will be able to understand the dynamics entailed in working with this kind of patient. However, a therapist that can be easily manipulated into giving the highly focused attention this type of patient craves would probably be most likely to gain the patient's patronage and, to a certain measure, his loyalty and trust. Though these patients may be likely to stay longest with therapists who fulfill their desires, the therapist who does this won't really be able to be effective as a therapist.

Jasmine: The Lonely Patient

Jasmine was a woman in her sixties: wealthy, well educated, and highly intelligent. She was also an accomplished poet and cellist, and her name occasionally decorated the society pages. She had been divorced twice and was estranged from three of her four children. She inserted herself into various social groups, ranging from a book group, to a musical society, to a group of "ladies who lunch." Since most of these people rarely spent more than an hour or two a month in her company, they weren't too put off by the fact that she totally dominated their get-togethers.

Jasmine liked to give very extravagant dinner parties to which she generally invited an intellectual or artistic crowd, including those from a nearby university. She paid an inordinate amount of attention to her clothing, food, flowers, and house furnishings, though her bedroom, which no one ever saw (she confided to her therapist), resembled a monk's cell. She professed to be very happy because she had so many friends and people who cared for her.

However, without understanding why, she was also extremely frightened at times, and this prompted her to seek therapy. She began therapy with a colleague of mine, Dr. N., but it only lasted for six sessions. In that brief time, Jasmine told Dr. N. how she had been victimized by her entire family, but unwittingly revealed to him that she had put a lot of energy into creating discord between family members with her repeated demands that she be the center of attention.

Jasmine viewed each person she came into contact with as someone who would either contribute to her happiness by making her feel special, or not. Unfortunately, the "not" included Dr. N., from whom Jasmine demanded unwavering adulation. She brought him expensive gifts the first three or four times they met (which he promptly refused); several times she claimed to have developed new and unusual symptoms and demanded he investigate them; and she called him several times between each session to make sure he was "focusing on her case." Dr. N. was highly motivated to treat Jasmine, not only because of his professional dedication, but also out of compassion. He had worked with people who had this type of disorder in the past and found the work challenging but rewarding.

During the sixth session with Jasmine, Dr. N. began to gently speak about Jasmine's challenges in sustaining relationships; it was his first attempt at pointing out where Jasmine might want to more deeply explore and understand her feelings and behaviors. Suddenly she stood up, told him that "he was not able to help her because he obviously didn't like her," and walked out the door. Dr. N. wasn't surprised, just saddened.

The next week Dr. N. followed up with Jasmine on the phone, as he did with all his former patients, just to make sure she was doing okay. She gushingly told him she had finally found the right therapist for her and, in fact, was going for a weeklong, one-on-one intensive therapy vacation in the British Virgin Islands with her new therapist. In other words, Jasmine had met her match—a so-called therapist (the therapist was not credentialed or licensed) who was able to beat Jasmine at her own game and make her pay for a Caribbean vacation for two.

Patients like Jasmine can be described as being very lonely without actually understanding what loneliness is.

A skilled therapist should be able to gauge what type of personality issues patients like Jasmine have and follow specific protocol in order to help them change. People might find patients with histrionic (and other) personality disorders uncomfortable to be around, but if properly motivated and treated, many can change over time.

Sometimes people facing these challenges won't seek therapy in order to change so much as to confirm that they are "better than okay" and that the problem is everybody else. Most of the time, though, these types of patients cause a kind of fallout. They don't end up in therapy, but the people who are in close contact with them (such as employees, spouses, and, most especially, their children), do. These fallout patients are stuck in the orbit of the person who has the personality disorder. They are bombarded by the space junk caused by that person's erratic, confusing, and hurtful behavior. The star may be sick, but it's the planets that usually end up seeking treatment.

And even if someone who has a severe personality disorder is actually motivated to change, the process will be exceedingly difficult and painful—and slow. One of the most difficult things for patients like this is to accept responsibility for their own thoughts, feelings, and behaviors. Anything negative that occurs is always someone else's fault; anything positive is their own doing. Most likely, if you are able to read through this chapter without becoming infuriated, this type of personality disorder is not your problem. However, we have included this rather extreme, real-life archetypal example of a patient like this because it might be beneficial to those readers who have family members who have been diagnosed with a personality disorder. We believe it is important that you become aware of several ways in which a patient might sabotage therapy and recognize this potential in those you love and even in yourself, if necessary.

Therapy Addiction

Another way a patient (sometimes with the collusion of or manipulation by his therapist) can thwart success in therapy is by becoming addicted to therapy. That is, he becomes addicted to the actual *type* of relationship—the relationship between therapist and patient. Or he becomes addicted to a particular therapist.

Therapy addiction fulfills all the criteria for a very real addiction. Just as an addiction to drugs, alcohol, gambling, food, and so on makes the patient feel as if he cannot live without the thing he craves, an addiction to therapy does the same. If you feel you may fit this description, talk about it with your therapist. But beware—if he has helped to facilitate your addiction in any way, perhaps by confusing boundaries or allowing or encouraging endless therapy, then speak about your concerns with someone else you trust and respect. That person may be a therapist, spiritual advisor, teacher, family member, or friend. Remember, your therapist should work hard to engage you in therapy, but not to the point of addiction.

The Fake-out

You dutifully go to therapy. You and your therapist agree upon a course of action while in the office. But once you leave, you don't do what the therapist recommends and what you have both agreed on. This patient fake-out is very common in therapy with those with eating disorders, gambling, and other behavioral addictions, as well as those with substance abuse or addiction.

Brenda's Attempted Fake-out

Brenda, a thirty-five-year-old nurse, had been referred to my program by a state disciplinary program that monitors nurses. She was mandated to complete a course of addiction treatment. Brenda had been diverting medications, mostly opiates, from the patients in the hospital where she worked and taking them herself. She also forged doctors' orders and even created phony patient charts in order to be able to requisition medications to feed her addiction.

My recommendations, though not absolute requirements in this case, included her attendance at the self-help meetings of her choice. I asked her to try out these "sober activities" and see if they could be of help to her. Many, though not all addicts find the incredibly supportive atmosphere of Alcoholics Anonymous, Narcotics Anonymous, and other 12-step programs to be a tremendous stepping-stone toward recovery. There are also special professional support groups, such as those for doctors or nurses, that can be helpful. There are even women-only groups and many more specialized types of meetings. Additionally, the state disciplinary agency that referred Brenda also had support groups she could have chosen to attend. Clearly, there were many options.

> *During the first few weeks of treatment, both in group and indi-*
> *vidual therapies, Brenda told me she was following my recommenda-*
> *tions. Actually, she wasn't. When I saw progress wasn't being made, I*
> *queried her about her support group meetings and she admitted that she*
> *hadn't been truthful before. She hadn't been attending any 12-step or*
> *other support groups. She argued that she would rather get the support*
> *of friends than go to a support group.*

It is true that sometimes a patient can choose a different objective than the therapist would choose, and it could be beneficial. In Brenda's case though, choosing to talk with her drug-using friends about her addiction was a poor choice. It was a way for her to thwart treatment. She was afraid to really give *recovery* a chance, and so her "methods" failed—because they were designed to fail. Recovery, in terms of psychotherapy and addiction treatment, happens when a person begins to make better choices about his physical, mental, or spiritual health. These are important areas in which recovery usually must take place. After a few months of therapy, Brenda finally overcame her fears and developed the requisite motivation to begin real recovery, in all the areas of her life. She began to attend support group meetings and today is committed to living a drug-free life.

Switching Seats on the *Titanic*

A commonly used phrase in the addiction recovery movement, the political world, and even the sports world is "switching seats on the *Titanic*." The classic example is someone who is addicted to alcohol and begins smoking marijuana instead of drinking; he is "switching seats" on a sinking ship. He is going to drown anyway. The phrase can sometimes apply to other therapy saboteurs, especially in the area of unhealthy behaviors, habits, or compulsions—

or anything else that is used to avoid correcting the root of a problem. If yelling at your spouse has endangered your marriage, don't switch seats on the *Titanic* and yell at your coworkers.

Switcheroo

You show up late or not at all. You refuse to talk about the important issues or ask to change your treatment plan every session. You offer unconvincing excuses or hem and haw. Perhaps you just tell your therapist you won't follow his recommendations. You decide you want to change the modality of therapy—for example, agree to only go to individual therapy, though group therapy is the recommended option, or vice versa. It may seem pointless for a patient to attend therapy then obstruct the course of therapy so blatantly, but it does happen on occasion. Some patients do "switch" on and off.

Far more common is that a *partner* in therapy is facilitating the switcheroo. Sometimes this therapy partner is a spouse; often it is a parent or legal guardian. Partners who are family members usually do want therapy to succeed—they love their sibling, spouse, or child. They are probably trying to be supportive. However, when a patient who is a child or spouse starts to get better, it often threatens the family system that is already in place, one that has operated the same way for years. This can trigger a lot of ambivalence in therapy partners. When a patient starts to improve, family roles will begin to shift, and this causes a very real period of upheaval.

In her book *Another Chance: Hope and Health for the Alcoholic Family*, therapist Sharon Wegscheider-Cruse describes the roles played by family members and gives them names such as the "mascot," the "superhero," and so on. When one person emerges from an old role, his liberation can cause a domino effect that is felt by the whole family. Now everyone has to change. Sometimes, for a variety of reasons, members of a family resist change, like Pam.

Pam: Resisting Change

A few years ago the principal of a private high school sent me a patient, a boy of about fifteen. Luke had some learning disabilities and had been accurately diagnosed (by being thoroughly tested several times) with attention deficit/hyperactivity disorder (ADHD). He also had severe emotional problems. The school was made up of a very dedicated team of educators who asked that the parents send Luke to any other therapist that met with their approval. In fact, they made his attendance at therapy twice a week a condition for allowing him to remain enrolled in the school.

I saw Luke for a few sessions. His situation really touched my heart. He exhibited signs of post-traumatic stress disorder, but we never got far enough along in therapy for me to diagnosis him with complete accuracy.

Luke's father was not involved in his son's education or therapy. He was a stern disciplinarian, rarely speaking to his son unless to punish him. He loved Luke but found it difficult to show it. He felt things were fine with Luke just the way they were and didn't want to hear about or participate in his therapy.

Luke's mother, Pam, was very involved in her son's life—in fact, it was she who chose this special school for him. She adored Luke and invested a tremendous amount of energy in parenting him. She wanted him to improve, to be happy, and to remain in this high school and graduate, but she bitterly resented the school dictating the terms of Luke's enrollment, that is, his participation in therapy. Unfortunately, she allowed her displeasure at having to relinquish control to taint her behavior. She blindly worked against her and Luke's best interests.

Pam did many things to thwart Luke's success. She rescheduled each therapy appointment several times; she refused to allow Luke to follow my recommendations; she would call to cancel appointments right when her son was due to arrive in my office. I had encouraged Luke to spend time playing sports to relieve tension; I (and his teachers) also encouraged him to join one of the many after-school clubs the school offered. His mother refused to allow him to participate in either the sports or the clubs.

After a couple of months went by, Pam's resistance escalated, despite constant phone meetings I scheduled with her. Luke's school counselor and I wanted to include Pam in the development of Luke's treatment plan, but she would change the subject whenever it was broached. She began to say that Luke was too "sick" to change and that he would never change. Then an emotional bomb went off. Luke's teachers and principal told Pam that they had to transfer Luke into classes more suited to his academic level—he was doing poorly in the classes he was in. They told her Luke was completely unable to keep up with his coursework, and this was contributing to his low self-esteem and depression. Pam was enraged and refused to give her permission for the switch.

She also refused to pay for tuition or treatment. I still agreed to treat Luke and told Pam that I would see him for free because I felt at this point Luke would have a painful setback if I stopped seeing him. When I spoke with the school, they felt it was in Luke's best interests to keep him on for the next semester despite the lack of payment and used special scholarship funds for his tuition. When she realized that she was not able to control the school, Pam demanded that I not coordinate

*his treatment with his teachers or school counselor. I refused to do this;
it was the only time I insisted on anything in Luke's treatment. I
explained to Pam that the only way for Luke to improve would be for
his teachers, counselor, and me to coordinate his care.*

*This didn't sit well with Pam, so she decided to withdraw Luke
from the school. She called me to tell me she was putting him in a res-
idential drug and alcohol treatment program, despite the fact that he
was not a substance abuser. He now would work with a private tutor
in the residence. She also asked me to continue treating him without
pay. I agreed but strongly urged her to reconsider withdrawing him
from the school, believing that this measure was not only utterly unnecessary but would totally undermine Luke's very fragile sense of self-
worth. Pam then told me that Luke was not allowed to see me
anymore. That was the last his teachers or I heard from Pam.*

*Today, Luke is in his twenties. Sometimes he lives at his parents'
home, sometimes on the streets. Don't let this be your kid.*

The Street Fight/Sucker Punch

Related to, and sometimes used in conjunction with the switcheroo is
what I call the *street fight*. In the street fight, the patient is usually deeply
afraid of rejection or being hurt by others, so he lashes out in order to pre-
empt any possible attacks. From this patient's perspective, it is hurt or be
hurt. There are no other options.

When street fighting, the patient manufactures arguments or disagree-
ments with the therapist. He may use vulgarities or attack the therapist in
an aggressive, provocative manner. Sometimes, the therapist will feel forced
to end contact with an abusive patient. When that happens, the patient
can then blame the therapist. "My therapist kicked me out." Because many

of the patients in treatment programs are volatile, this is not such unusual behavior. The therapists who work with me are trained to cope with this behavior, minimize the attacks, and keep the patient in therapy—unless he is a danger to himself or others. If he is, we help him get more appropriate care.

One of the tactics of a street fight is the *sucker punch*. The sucker punch can only happen when a victim's guard is down and his opponent also knows the victim's weak spots. For example, I have a colleague who is a devout Christian. Though she is a highly professional addiction therapist and is well able to keep religion out of therapy discussions, she informs her patients of her beliefs in case they would prefer to find another therapist. Every now and then she will get a patient who sabotages therapy with a sucker punch. The patient will tell her he has just participated in an act that most people, let alone a religious Christian, would find offensive, such as an illegal act or particularly wild personal exploits. Because she knows that these kinds of attacks are manufactured to push her to end therapy, she is always prepared to work through them with the patient if they occur.

Therapists who do not come across this kind of aggressive, sabotaging behavior frequently may be at a loss in how to deal with it. No wonder. It can be frightening. Let me advocate for therapists here (and advocate for you to remain in therapy when you need to): don't pick a fight with your therapist!

You Don't Know How It Feels

You are right! Your therapist can't possibly know how it really feels to have (take your pick): depression, addiction, bipolar disorder, post-traumatic stress disorder, and so on (unless he has had them himself). He has no idea what it feels like to be you. No one is able to really know what that's like.

On the one hand, a therapist doesn't need to have felt what you are feeling, whether it is a craving for alcohol or a blind rage, in order to treat you. But if a therapist, or any person for that matter, has had similar experiences or similar emotions, it feels somehow easier for us to trust his advice. When we are suffering and we are able to speak with someone else who really understands what we feel like, we feel validated. But keep in mind, *a thera-pist doesn't have to know how you feel to know how to heal*.

Like a heart surgeon who doesn't have to have heart disease to do a bypass, a therapist doesn't have to have your particular problem to treat it. The surgeon understands the workings of the heart, veins, arteries, valves, and so on. He understands how to use his scalpel and how to suture. He knows how to prevent infection. A therapist has had training in the way the mind and emotions operate. He has learned, practiced, and seen recovery happen with a variety of techniques.

In actuality, though, your therapist has had some shared experiences that help him personally relate to at least part of what you are going through, unlike the physical problems a physician might never be able to share with his patient. A therapist has feelings, emotions, and thoughts that are, in many important ways, like your own. Most human beings, including your therapist, share a capacity for suffering, joy, anxiety, calmness, love, hate, anger, and forgiveness. We may not know exactly how others are feeling, but we all have probably felt something along the spectrum of others' emotional experiences. In part because of this a therapist will be able to reach out to you with great compassion and enter into—and help you improve—your emo-tional world. It's a cop-out to say he isn't able to understand.

It may be helpful to know that everyone has had feelings along the same spectrum, if not at the same point, that you've had. We can create an imag-inary spectrum of an emotional problem, say, anxiety (see Figure 8.1). We can see that most people—including people who aren't currently facing emo-tional or mental problems—have experienced some form of anxiety at some point along this spectrum. That goes for psychotherapists, too.

Figure 8.1
Emotional Spectrum: Anxiety

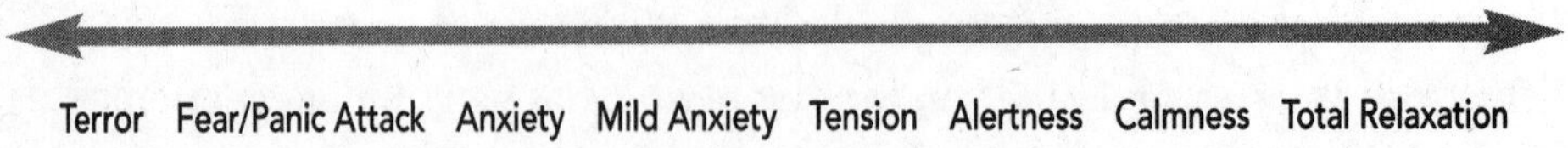

Terror   Fear/Panic Attack   Anxiety   Mild Anxiety   Tension   Alertness   Calmness   Total Relaxation

We can do the same thing with the symptoms of addiction. (Figure 8.2):

Figure 8.2
Symptom Spectrum: Addiction

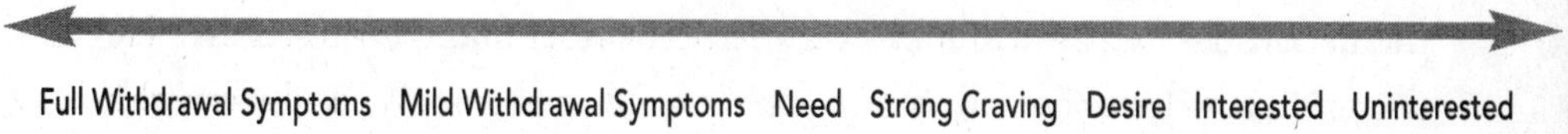

$$\longleftrightarrow$$

Full Withdrawal Symptoms   Mild Withdrawal Symptoms   Need   Strong Craving   Desire   Interested   Uninterested

Many emotional, mental, and even physical problems can be put onto a spectrum. You might want to ask your psychotherapist to help you create a spectrum to explore the full range of your feelings and emotions.

Staring into the Rearview Mirror

You are driving down a bumpy, two-lane country road on a rainy day. A gale is blowing and has knocked a couple of large branches into your path. Potholes are a constant hazard as are deer that seem to fly onto the road out of nowhere. There are cars in front of you that are going under the speed limit. What do you do? You keep your eyes on the road, glancing occasionally into the rearview mirror to see what's behind you. That is the way most therapy should be approached as well. You move forward, paying attention to the difficulties right ahead and a bit farther down the road, while just checking in with the past. What you shouldn't do is stare into the rearview mirror (your past), without giving any attention to what's ahead. Otherwise, you'll crash.

However, you may need to check into your past at least briefly. You may even need to spend some time talking about it. It may help you put the pieces of the puzzle—that is you—together. And if your past has so traumatized you that you can't remember or talk about it, it might take some time, perhaps several months or longer, to approach the subject and work through it. But neglecting the present and the future in order to immerse yourself in the past can cause you to lose perspective and avoid responsibility for who you are now and who you want to be tomorrow. Sometimes patients and their therapists return again and again to the past in order to dredge up negative experiences, kind of like the way your tongue goes to that sore tooth despite the fact that every time you touch it, it hurts.

The past will come up in therapy again and again, but past events, even if negative, should be mined for whatever positives can be gleaned from them. Because there are linkages between the present and the past, of course you and your therapist will want to understand your past. *While understanding the past is important, it is more important to avoid getting stuck in it.*

It is also important to not look too far into the future but to deal with what is going on in the present. My advice to most of you: *Let's peek at the past, stay in the present, and prepare for the future.* Or, in the words made immortal by Oogway in the movie *Kung Fu Panda,* "Yesterday is history. Tomorrow is a mystery. Today is a gift. That's why we call it the present." Remember, most of the time the present is where our minds and hearts belong.

Dishonesty Is the Worst Policy

If you are keeping a therapy journal, you might want to keep a log of how you may be blocking or sabotaging treatment and talk it over with your therapist. There are different levels of awareness, but if you and your therapist work on paying attention to what feelings, emotions, and thoughts you are experiencing in the present, you will be able to become more aware if you are sabotaging your progress. You will also fine-tune your sense of honesty and integrity—something that can benefit everyone.

Chapter 9

TRACKING PROGRESS

All truths are easy to understand once they are discovered;
the point is to discover them.

—GALILEO GALILEI

It's safe to say one of the main goals of therapy is to teach you how to help yourself so you don't actually have to be in therapy, at least not for a moment longer than necessary. When you have made the changes you set out to make, both you and your therapist will then take a closer look and see if it is time for you to move on.

How do you recognize that you have made these changes? The first step is, once again, to create a treatment plan at the beginning of therapy and to refer to it throughout. Your treatment plan will help you to isolate behaviors, feelings, or thoughts that you want to change. Then the listed objectives and goals may be held as the standards by which your therapeutic achievements can be measured. If your treatment plan is comprehensive, you will find it far easier to make both objective and subjective assessments about your progress. Without a treatment plan as the starting point, it will be challenging if not

impossible to accurately measure improvements, kind of like trying to measure out a cup of water in an old boot. If you have no parameters or measures,
you will inevitably be way off the mark.

How to Recognize Positive Change

Questions must be asked to determine if you did indeed make the necessary changes called for in your treatment plan, such as "Did I achieve Objective A?" and "Has Goal B become a part of my life?" There are other essential
questions you need to ask about your progress. Your therapist and you should
touch base and answer questions like the following many times over the
course of therapy:

- Do I have longer and longer periods of maintaining positive changes?
  (For example, if you are depressed and your goal is to move from recognizing and experiencing the symptoms of depression to managing
  depression, you may measure your success by asking if either the
  duration of your depression or the severity of it have lessened.)
- Have these changes happened within a reasonable treatment time
  frame?
- Is there additional progress that may not be listed on the treatment
  plan that my therapist or I have observed? What is it?
- Have I developed the skills I need to manage the problems in my life
  with minimal support, that is, without regular therapy sessions?

There are also other methods that can help you, over time, keep track of
your progress. If appropriate, your therapist may ask you to rate your progress
regarding your feelings, thoughts, and behaviors. This can help you more
closely measure your therapeutic achievements. Let's say your therapist asks
you to rate feelings of anxiety on a scale of 1 to 10, with 10 being the most
extreme and 1 being no anxiety at all—a state of total calmness. You may be
asked to use this system to rate your feelings as they occur under various stressors. By becoming aware when anxiety is mounting, for example, and by
learning techniques to manage the anxiety before it spirals out of control, you

should notice that your "ratings" begin to go down—which is a good thing! Therefore, if you begin therapy with an anxiety rating of 9 when coping with stressful situations, and over time you have worked your way down to a 3 or 4, you have made measurable and real progress. This system is designed to function in the structure of a popular operational model called "pre-test, test, and post-test."

A less definitive but deeper way to understand and recognize positive change is to develop a greater personal awareness of your feelings, thoughts, and behaviors. Ultimately, this will help you understand who you are and what you need to do so you can continue to grow and improve. Your therapist should help you accomplish this by recommending one or more methods—including a therapy journal and/or the PPP mentioned in Chapter 6. By learning how to articulate your thoughts and feelings, recording them either on paper or on audio- or videotape, and analyzing them, you will become more aware over time. As you become more aware, you will recognize the changes you have made and begin to understand their implications at a deeper level. You will also be better able to replicate methods that lead to positive change.

Questions that will help you recognize change at a deeper level, and that can be explored in sessions, through your journal, or in a PPP might include:

- Do I reflect more positively about traumatic situations in my life than I did in the past?
- Do I more often feel at peace?
- Am I better able to manage negative feelings and respond to life's challenges with courage and optimism?
- Do I feel "together" for more sustained periods of time (could be hours, days, weeks, or months depending on where you started)?
- Am I more frequently able to understand the consequences of my behavior/actions and do these potential consequences influence my behavior/actions in advance?
- Am I more frequently able to put myself in others' shoes and also not *personalize* (incorrectly take another's remarks or actions as applying to myself) their actions?

The questions above are only suggestions. Your therapist will help you develop questions and answers that will reflect your specific, personal needs.

Chatting Versus Directed Discussions

Many patients do see improvements in therapy (they become less angry, less depressed, etc.), but the progress happens over tremendously long periods of time. Remember Lisa from Chapter 7? She reported that over time—five years—she became less angry. That change may have occurred far sooner with a tighter, more determined therapeutic focus.

A patient who recently consulted with me had been in therapy for nine years with the same therapist. He told me that after several years, he found it easier to be assertive (his primary goal) than when he started therapy, but he wasn't sure it was worth the cost of nine years of therapy! He said most of the time he felt like he was just "chatting" with his therapist. He is not the only patient that I have heard describe his therapy experience this way.

I don't want to negate the importance of *talking*—either with friends or therapists. It is good to talk. However, *chatting* is directionless talk, and therapy requires direction, focus, and commitment. Chatting might be fine when it's done with friends or acquaintances or very early on in therapy when your therapist and you are beginning to cultivate your relationship. But remember, you are paying your therapist for an exclusive, specific, and professional service. Your time is valuable, too.

Simply put, one of your therapist's main jobs is to help *accelerate* your recovery. Perhaps over time and with a bevy of self-help books, you could find your way to wellness without therapy—many people have. But it shouldn't take so long with the help of a good therapist.

Clinical excellence and reasonable speed of treatment can go hand in hand. Some schools of therapy have a different approach, and speedy recovery is not a focus of their outlook. I believe—and many therapists agree—tangible results that occur in a reasonable time frame are more important than adherence to an elite therapeutic ideal. The speedy relief of suffering and the ability to help a patient begin to live a fuller life trump loyalty to a therapeutic philosophy. To me and many therapists this is a moral imperative.

Also, I feel that the ability of some long-term clinical approaches to effect change (such as psychoanalysis) is questionable. After all, people change over time whether or not they are in therapy—they mature, develop insights into themselves and others, and even improve their behavior. In his book *Generation to Generation: Personal Recollections of a Chassidic Legacy* respected psychiatrist Rabbi Abraham J. Twerski, M.D., writes of the time when he considered practicing psychoanalysis. His father pointed out to him that treatment that takes such a long time as psychoanalysis will naturally coincide with changes in a patient. "You are going to treat a patient for several years and then claim that your treatment helped him? Just think of how many things can happen in those years that may alter his life situation for the better. He may find a new job, he may marry, he may divorce, he may move away from meddling in-laws, his enemies may die, he may have children. Why, there is no limit to the kinds of things that may transpire during a period of several years. How can you take credit for his improvement?"

Rabbi Doctor Twerski says, "To me, this made good sense. I embraced brief psychotherapy long before the insurance companies mandated it."

If your therapist works with you strategically and economically—driven by your goals and their target dates—the rate at which you reach those goals will be accelerated. There is every reason to think you will become less dependent on therapy. In order to make the most of those precious therapy minutes, tightly focused sessions are the order of the day.

Problem Solving

As you assess your therapy experience, you will want to gauge whether or not you have been able to apply what you have learned to your life. You must make these new ways of living your own, embracing them daily. That may mean practicing techniques your therapist gives you, such as anger management techniques, over and over again, until they become second nature. Or it may mean writing copiously in your therapy journal and reflecting on what is written there. Or actively thinking about how to solve problems and developing step-by-step plans to do so. Or charting your progress in minute detail and paying attention to which techniques work— and which don't.

Whatever recommendations your therapist makes, they will be based on *reproductive* and *productive problem solving*. Reproductive problem solving is using what you know already, or have already experienced, to make positive change happen. Productive problem solving is using new ideas to make positive change happen.

When you allow yourself to see links between the present and the past, and develop the skills needed to examine and understand those links and make appropriate changes, you will be doing reproductive problem solving. The next time you encounter similar situations, you will respond in an improved manner. In effect, you are recycling the past, taking what appears to have nothing to offer and turning it into something useful, perhaps even beautiful.

For example, let's suppose that last week you became furious when someone cut in front of you in line at the grocery store, and the day before yesterday you became enraged when someone cut you off in traffic. And today, right before your therapy appointment, you were told you didn't get a job you applied for and you became angry. When you arrive at your appointment, you let loose and tell your therapist how ticked off you are.

Your therapist may begin by trying to help you see similarities between these events. He may ask you to think about why they angered you. Could your anger be about your inability to control situations in your life? Could your anger be rooted in not "getting where you want to go" without encountering seemingly random obstacles? What do the obstacles really represent? You will most likely talk about these connections with your therapist. You may want to write down, tape-record, or otherwise note the connections between life's challenges and your responses to them. Over time you will learn how to see these challenges as personal growth opportunities, even spiritual opportunities. You may further recycle these events by mining them for deeply buried treasures. What do these events and your responses to them have to say about who you are?

In general, productive problem solving will at first be facilitated by your therapist. He should gently share with you new ways of understanding and solving your problems. He may say phrases like, "Have you ever thought of looking at X in this way?" Or, "Have you ever considered this possibility in relation to Y?" These unfamiliar ways of viewing problems will be supported by new skills your therapist will help you develop, and be able to use on your own at some point.

Sometimes productive problem solving can be a bit complicated, perhaps even mystical, because it can involve *sudden insights*. Sudden insights (or "aha experiences") are little-understood moments of deep comprehension that appear to spring up without the slow development and trial and error that is inherent in reproductive problem solving. However, it really doesn't have to be mysterious in the least. *A new outlook + the application of practical skills = goals met.*

Past events can help you find ways to deal with the future. You will use both reproductive and productive problem solving to create a plan to deal with problems on both emotional and practical levels. For example, suppose you find that when you are alone feelings of depression become magnified. In addition to finding the triggers that cause you to feel depressed, your therapist will help you actively resolve or manage symptoms, or develop healthy coping mechanisms.

Perhaps listening to music will help you avoid some periods of depression, or perhaps volunteering at a local hospital will better help you take the focus off your negative feelings. Maybe your therapist will suggest that when you are alone you can spend time in a creative endeavor such as writing poetry, cooking, or knitting, which, while not a "cure" can help you channel negative feelings in positive ways. Perhaps, temporarily, you have to limit contact with people who trigger negative feelings. Maybe antidepressants are required. Whatever the solutions, and there will usually be more than one possibility, trial and error are a large part of both reproductive and productive problem solving.

As you explore the nature of a problem itself, above and beyond just the solution to the problem, you will gain deeper insight. Let's return to our example of loneliness magnifying depression. The problem is depression. What lessons can be learned about *you* from the context in which your feelings of depression take place? In our example, that of being alone triggering symptoms of depression, the context in which the depression happens itself can indicate that there is work to be done. There might be a real need to either develop a greater ability to be independent or, conversely, learn how to reach out to others more. A dedicated therapist can help you further recycle your problem at many levels. He might suggest that you explore ways in which you can become more compassionate and understanding of others who are feeling depressed. Depending on how far you want to take it, a therapist might even suggest you teach others the problem-solving techniques you learn in therapy as a way in which to concretize your newfound skills.

Just hearing about or understanding therapeutic problem-solving techniques won't magically make your thoughts, feelings, and behaviors change. You must work hard to develop the skill sets (groups of skills) that will help facilitate those changes. After you practice these skills in real-life situations, you will most likely be asked to report back to your therapist on your experiences. Together you will analyze the events and note where you need to improve. This procedure should strengthen your commitment to change. Also, if your therapist is helping you develop skills in one area of your life, let's say improving your relationship with coworkers, he should also help you generalize those skills and apply them in other areas of life, such as by improving relationships with family members

Psychoeducation

Part of problem solving in general is gaining a thorough understanding of your problems and possible solutions to them. Therapists use *psychoeducation* to educate you (and your partners in therapy) about the problems or illnesses you are struggling with in order to help you (and your partners) understand what to expect from the illness and what treatment is required.

For example, if you are abusing alcohol, your therapist may explain to you the physiological and psychological effects of alcoholism, give you a reading list about the subject, and recommend you take a prevention class to further learn about abuse and addiction. If you are depressed, he may give you articles to read about depression, talk about its causes and how it affects behavior, explain treatment options, and even educate you about brain chemistry.

Another part of psychoeducation is learning strategies to deal with your problems. Using terms you can understand, your therapist will educate you about skills you can learn in order to manage your problems. For example, if a therapist tells you that you need to be more assertive, he is making a statement, not educating you. Without knowing why you need to be more assertive, and what the concept of assertiveness really means, you won't have the understanding to make healthy changes. To help you become more assertive, an experienced therapist may teach you about four types of communication:

- **Passive:** behaviors and/or ways of communicating that show little or no visible behavioral reaction (though there may be an internal reaction going on); verbal agreement with another even if internal disagreement exists.
- **Passive-aggressive:** behaviors and/or ways of communicating that express negative feeling such as resentment and aggression in a nonassertive and nonovertly aggressive way (may include procrastination, stubbornness, sullenness, and unwillingness to communicate).
- **Aggressive:** behaviors and/or ways of communicating that are verbally or physically violent or designed to harm another.
- **Assertive:** behaviors and/or ways of communicating that are self-assured, confident, and express how you are feeling. One of the important aspects of assertiveness is that you take "ownership" of your feelings, behaviors, and consequences. Also, genuine assertiveness is about communicating effectively.

He may *role-play* with you to help you understand the differences between them. Role-play involves acting out of a past or future event with the therapist assuming the role of one of the participants in the event, and the patient, the other. He may help you explore examples in your life when you have used these various types of communication and discuss the results of each. He may help you identify with whom and in what circumstances you are most likely to be passive, aggressive, and so on. If you are not easily able to identify the types of communication you engage in, more psychoeducation may be necessary. Also, more processing of past experiences may help you communicate more effectively.

Internalize and Apply

With effective therapy, the skill sets and lessons you learn will become an integral part of you and your life. You will internalize them; they will become second nature to you. You will also be able to apply these skills in a variety of situations. You may have to take baby steps, though—analyzing situations thoroughly and applying the skills you learn tentatively until you are more confident.

Internalize and apply is a slightly different process than *identify and apply*, as Laron from Chapter 6 first learned to do. Internalizing is the next step after identifying. When you identify a problem and apply a technique to address it, you are figuring out what the problem is and "trying out" a solution. When you internalize the technique, you are making that solution your own.

Remember Samantha, the interior designer in Chapter 6? Part of her struggle was with assertiveness. She had been attempting to control her employee, Rafael, in a mostly passive-aggressive manner. She used silence or deflection as a *defense mechanism* to assert her superiority. (Defense mechanism, as it is used here, refers to unconscious, negative psychological strategies brought into play by an individual in order to help him or her from experiencing specific, uncomfortable feelings; the following are examples of defense mechanisms: intellectualizing, generalizing, rationalizing, blaming, justifying, etc.).

She and I spoke about developing a healthier communication style, that of assertiveness. But when I asked her to role-play with me and show me what assertive communication meant, she acted aggressively, yelling and bullying. She hadn't yet learned the difference between assertiveness and aggression. Together we worked on helping her understand what assertiveness really was.

Perhaps Samantha, in an attempt to be assertive, would have become openly hostile to Rafael if she and I hadn't role-played first. Fortunately, she was able to apply what she learned in therapy. Now she could be assertive when necessary, and her relationship with Rafael dramatically improved as a consequence. After time, she became comfortable enough to also appropriately apply her assertiveness skills when she spoke with her sister, her mother, and others. Most of her relationships and the feelings she had about these relationships began to improve.

You will know problem solving, psychoeducation, internalizing, and applying are truly working when your use of the skills you learned in therapy have become so automatic that you barely notice you are using them. You will begin to deal far more effectively with life's challenges. People will respond to you differently, and your relationships will improve.

Whatever the methods used to get to the point where you have internalized and applied the lessons of psychotherapy, *internalize and apply* is an apt description of the nature of *all* therapy gains. In Chapter 10, we will continue to discuss internalizing and applying after you leave therapy.

Time, Context, Experience

You might specifically come to therapy to make sense of painful, traumatic, or shameful events in your past. You may feel these events are still affecting you. By allowing yourself to acknowledge and explore the links between your present and your past, you will see your life in a new light. Or, exploring past events may be something you decide to do after coming to therapy for a different reason. (Remember, though, therapy doesn't have to be about the past; just focusing on the present is an excellent choice for many people.) Asking and answering the following three types of questions about past events—placing them in *time*, in the *context* in which they happened, and your *experience* of the events—will help you integrate your past experiences into a healthier future.

1. The Time Question

When did the event in question happen? How old was I? Was I three or was I ten? How many years ago was that? An event is locked in time—we can't go back and change it. As we get older, we may be able to look back on the event with more mature vision. However, sometimes our vision is also locked in time. If an event is traumatizing, or very painful, we might still remember it and react to it as if we were the age during which the event happened.

For example, if at nine years old you were a victim of a violent crime, when recalling it, you might still react as if you were nine years old again. By first assigning the correct time and age at the start of any discussion about an event and how old you feel when you remember it, you will gain insight into how you perceived the event then (and how you view it now).

2. The Context Question

What was going on before, during, and after in the time and place in which the event occurred? Where did the event occur? What was going on around me before, during, and after its occurrence? What were the people involved in the event— including me—doing that led up to the event? What did we do afterward? What else happened after the event?

For example, remember where you were before the attack occurred. You were walking down your street in the late afternoon. It was almost dark. You were nearly at your house. Suddenly, a group of adolescents from another neighborhood appeared and started taunting you. They were shouting racial epithets. You froze. The boys then began to push you, and one grabbed your book bag and hit you with it. They stole your schoolbooks and your allowance money. They also humiliated you, calling you names. They beat you severely enough so that you needed stitches in your head and face. Afterward you ran home, but no one was there. Your parents were out. You tried to stop the bleeding and then finally called 911. You went to the hospital, and your parents, who had both been at work, showed up a few hours later.

By describing the event in detail a few times, it becomes more manage-able and loses a lot of its power over you. If others were involved in an upset-ting event, their motivations may even be discussed. Viewing others as flawed, sick, or ignorant, rather than viewing them as all-powerful monsters, might also be helpful to you. Even if the event didn't involve others, break-ing it down into manageable parts can minimize negative feelings.

3. The Experience Question

What was my internal experience of the event, then and now? What were/are my feelings about what happened? What did it really feel like to be me at the time, and how does it feel now to remember it? How did my age, my awareness, or the context in which the event happened limit my understanding of the event?

In our imaginary example, during the event you felt alternately terrified and ashamed. You were also in physical pain. You felt abandoned when your parents didn't show up at the hospital right away, even though you under-stood they couldn't be reached. Afterward you became afraid of walking home from school. You waited at school until your parents could pick you up on their way home after work until the end of the school year. Even now, just thinking about it makes you feel shame. You are still scared of walking alone sometimes, and even small groups of adolescent boys still scare you. When outside your house, you feel as if you are almost constantly on edge and are hypervigilant. You would like to work on that hypervigilance and learn to relax and trust that you are safe.

Of course, an incident like the one described above is a dramatic event that would traumatize many people, but not all would have the same reac-tions to it. As you explore the events that make up your life, you will also be exploring how the events have helped shape who you are, both positively and negatively. This will lead to the development of insight over time, rather than the flash of sudden insight we spoke about earlier. Also, dissecting and analyzing the event's aftereffects can help you develop the skills needed to see the positive potential in seemingly negative events.

In our example, you may come to realize this attack led you to actively seek out friendships with children who weren't racist. Perhaps all those hours spent waiting at school for your parents to pick you up led to you joining an after-school science club, which led you to your career in science. Maybe your parents began to take you to karate lessons, which improved your coordination and confidence. Now you want to work on your feelings of anxiety and hypervigilance, but you can see that the event triggered positive outcomes as well.

Transforming Status and Transcending Labels

A *label* is a narrow, one-dimensional term used as an all-encompassing description that severely restricts understanding. If believed in, a label has the power to determine status or a person's position in relationship to others. When you refuse to continue to be defined by a label, or when you genuinely feel that there has been a positive change in your status, you will know that progress is being made. Here are two experiences that illustrate this point.

Jennifer and Adam: Getting Out of "Victimhood"

Jennifer viewed herself as a victim of her parents. True, they didn't have the kind of parenting skills that would have encouraged stability, and sometimes they crossed the line into emotional abuse. As a small girl Jennifer alternated between states of all-encompassing grief and explosive frustration. As an adult she began retreating into a state of permanent victimhood and spent the majority of her life (she was fifty) seeking confirmation from everyone that she was, indeed, a lifelong victim. She continued to blame her parents for her failings, as well as others in her life. Naturally, this caused problems in many of her relationships.

Slowly her therapist, Melanie, began working with her on differentiating between having been a helpless child in the past and being an adult responsible for her own actions in the present. They problem solved and processed the events in Jennifer's childhood. Jennifer learned techniques to manage her anger and frustration. She began to stop comparing herself to others; she realized that victimhood was a badge she wore to avoid dealing with relationships, to avoid being hurt, and to shirk responsibility. Melanie helped her develop a rating system. That way Jennifer could recognize and monitor those times when she resorted to blaming others for her problems. Because she really wanted to change and worked hard to do so, over time Jennifer's view of herself underwent a dramatic transformation. Within a year, her status changed, and she rejected the limitations of labeling herself a victim.

Adam came to see me about depression. He told me that he had been sexually abused by a trusted teacher when he was six. As an eighteen-year-old college student, his life began spiraling out of control. He began drinking heavily and skipping classes. He was having many casual relationships that left him feeling very sad and ashamed. It took him several months of therapy to open up and share his traumatic childhood experience. For many years he felt responsible for his teacher's behavior. He secretly believed that it was his fault his teacher abused him and was greatly conflicted about what happened. In fact, he believed that he had "seduced" his teacher; after all, that was what his teacher had told him.

First, Adam had to get to the point where he understood that he had been a victim of a crime. For Adam, acknowledging that he had been a victim was a healthy first step. Unlike Jennifer, he needed to accept the limitations of status and label that victimhood conferred. In short, by accepting that he had been a victim, he was able to take the initial steps needed to release himself from the shackles of responsibility

> *for his teacher's criminal actions. Then he could begin to move beyond labels and learn to take responsibility for his present actions.*
>
> *During the course of intensive therapy, Adam's sense of his status had undergone major changes (from seducer, to victim, to neither). His status change, like Jennifer's, signaled that therapy had been effective.*

Your therapist should help you understand how status and labels can limit you. Although it might be important, as in Adam's case, to understand that you were a victim in the past or to learn that you have a disease such as schizophrenia or even for you to admit that you are an alcoholic, in general you and your therapist should avoid labels. Your therapist's job is to illustrate and describe, and to encourage *you* to illustrate and describe, not label.

Sometimes a diagnosis can become a label. While many people prefer to get an official "diagnosis" from a psychotherapist, I view a diagnosis as primarily necessary for insurance purposes, except perhaps in cases when it's important to educate a patient and his family about the illness he is facing. A diagnosis can sometimes lead therapists to miss vital clues to individual treatment paths. It is far more important for a therapist to get to know the person behind a diagnosis.

After all, your therapist doesn't really know you, at least not at first. Instead of labeling you a "victim," he might say something like, "It seems to me that you were really hurt by your husband when he yelled at you." Or instead of calling you a "help-rejecting complainer," he might say, "Perhaps in this and other instances you weren't ready to accept help when it was offered to you."

At no point should your therapist make leaping inferences about you— he could be wrong! He can't always presuppose that you feel or act a certain way because you fall into a diagnostic category. He has to do the groundwork to get to really know you as an individual.

In some cases your therapist might use what is called *advanced-level accu-*

rate empathy, that is, a tentative, educated estimate of what might be going on inside you. This is useful when patients have a difficult time communicating their feelings and thoughts. An example of advanced-level accurate empathy might be, "It seems to me you are a very caring person, but perhaps that quality, while generally an excellent one, has led you to not establish strong and healthy boundaries with others." By showing you some new ways to describe your inner world, your therapist will be setting an example for you to develop healthy insights. However, even though this is not labeling, this type of description should be used by your therapist only when needed. An important goal of therapy is to help you learn how to describe your inner world yourself, as well as transcend labels. Once you change your status and rise above labels, you can begin to take responsibility for who you are now and who you want to be.

Environmental Warrior

You also must take responsibility for where and with whom the positive changes you are making are to take place. If you are trying to stop drinking, and your roommate is an alcoholic, you live next door to a bar, and you craft ceramic beer mugs for a living, that is an environmental disaster waiting to happen. Your therapist may suggest you move out or find a new roommate. Perhaps he will suggest you use your pottery talents to make vases instead of beer mugs. If you want your environment to support the healthy new lifestyle you envision for yourself, changes may be required. And this doesn't just apply to addictions. Any mental or emotional problem may require practical changes.

If, for example, you have a social phobia (let's say you are painfully shy) and you do computer work from home, live in a remote rural cabin ten miles from the nearest neighbor, and your only roommate is your cat, you have an environmental problem. Your therapist should, at the right point in time, encourage you to make changes that will support your ability to create and sustain meaningful relationships. Perhaps he will encourage you to take a part-time job in a busy office, get a roommate, or do some people-oriented volunteer work. Maybe join a gym.

Remember though, one person's solution could be someone else's problem! An opposite situation could indeed exist. Maybe you never spend any time alone and you need to strengthen your independence in order to achieve your personal goals. With the support of your therapist, it can be possible to make whatever environmental changes are necessary in order to support the healthier lifestyle you want to have. *Taking responsibility for the choices you make about the people, places, and things in your life is an essential part of good therapy.*

Spirituality, Serenity, and Understanding

A therapeutic explanation of spirituality might go something like this: Any conceptualization or sequence of events that brings you closer to your highest potential relationship with yourself or others can be called a spiritual event. Anything that brings you closer to God and/or Good Orderly Direction and/or the higher power and/or the universal force can be called a spiritual event. Spirituality, or the way in which you actively choose to understand these events in your life and apply the lessons you have learned from them in a positive, growth-oriented way, helps you frame the broad variety of life experiences in a meaningful way and helps you uncover the essence of who you are.

Though spirituality is thought to blossom in religious disciplines, it can also achieve a toehold in the secular world. There are some religious disciplines that state that bliss and personal inner peace are the ultimate in spirituality, while some secular ideals base a kind of spiritual culture on personal moral responsibility for one's thoughts, speech, and actions. Clearly, the latter is far more developed ethically than the former, despite its lack of connection to a religion. We would further argue that the kind of "me first" emotional hedonism that passes for spirituality in some quasi-religious cultures today is actually very damaging to the self.

We want to emphasize that if you aren't open to any discussion of spirituality, you will be limiting yourself. By pushing aside or ignoring an essential part of what it means to be a human being, you will not be able to get a "multidimensional picture" of human life in general, and a multidimensional picture of your life in particular. Acknowledging that life has many levels, some unseen, reminds us of the switch from drab black-and-white Kansas to the Technicolor land of Oz in the classic movie, *The Wizard of Oz*. Dorothy the heroine can't really know or appreciate who she is or know and appreciate the people in her life until she experiences and explores Oz, a metaphorical version of her world back home. Integrating the rich lessons she learns in Oz with her life back home, Dorothy enters "recovery."

The spiritual starting point in recovery for people who are mentally ill or addicted is often one of deficit, that is, spiritual bankruptcy. That starting point suggests that just beginning to move in a direction that gets you closer to your potential best relationship with the world is the first step.

For people who aren't mentally ill or addicted, but are in therapy to work on less-overwhelming mental or emotional problems, that first step might be higher up the ladder—perhaps you want to explore more about the deeper meaning of your life or how you can align yourself with positive action. Relating to your own highest power might be a starting point for you. Or, your starting point might openly be about your relationship with God. We believe that any discussion of spirituality, no matter how basic, is essential to therapy.

But, please note: Unless you are specifically and purposefully seeking counsel from a therapist in order to help you do therapy work in a religious context, your therapist should not lead you in the direction of a specific religion. He may suggest that he help you begin to explore your foundational values and your spirituality—and if you feel his viewpoints are aligned with yours in basic ways, go ahead. Many, if not most psychotherapists do feel that understanding the complete person requires discussion of this uniquely human quality called spirituality.

Relinquishing Control

The very next thing you can do after taking responsibility for your environment, thoughts, feelings, and actions is to learn to relinquish some control. That sounds like a counterintuitive and even paradoxical course of action, but it is a very important step. Relinquishing control does not mean relinquishing personal responsibility—it means recognizing that you are not always able to control events. You are only able to control (at least most of the time!) yourself. For some people, relinquishing control may have to come before taking responsibility; for others, taking personal responsibility for what is in your control may have to be the first step. Together you and a skilled therapist will be able to determine what your priorities are.

By accepting that there are limits on your ability to control everything, you will begin to come closer to understanding what your overarching life mission is. Like the Rolling Stones used to sing, "You can't always get what you want, but if you try sometimes, you might find, you get what you need." Sometimes allowing things to happen and accepting the outcomes is a skill we all must learn.

This recognition can be humbling, but is essential to maturity. Seemingly negative events can even "conspire" to educate or enlighten you. Don't insist on total control or perfection—otherwise you will miss opportunities for growth.

Once you are able to recognize your own power limits, you should begin to recognize that you have a personal responsibility to improve what is in your power to do. This viewpoint has been condensed into a generalized prayer known as the "Serenity Prayer." It has been used by Alcoholics Anonymous and other 12-step programs, and most people have heard of it:

> GOD GRANT ME THE SERENITY
> TO ACCEPT THE THINGS I CANNOT CHANGE;
> COURAGE TO CHANGE THE THINGS I CAN;
> AND WISDOM TO KNOW THE DIFFERENCE.

This nondenominational prayer is not a substitute for, but an adjunct to your belief system. It acknowledges the existence of God and our relationship with him. If this is not comfortable for you, go ahead and instead acknowledge a universal higher power or even *the higher power of the best inner self you can possibly be.* You have to start from where you are "at" and not contort yourself into psychic pretzels to embrace any belief unless you are ready to do so. Your therapist shouldn't place demands on you to believe in something you aren't ready to believe in. And if you find difficulty with the concept of prayer in general, then go ahead and call it the "serenity affirmation" rather than the "Serenity Prayer."

The "Serenity Prayer" aptly describes what each and every individual's most fundamental, positive, psychospiritual goals should be: first, the ability to accept what we truly cannot change about ourselves, others, and the world. Next, we must understand there is a higher power at work in our lives. The prayer also posits that we should have the gumption and sense of personal responsibility to go inward (or reach outward) to make positive change—when we are able to do so.

Don't be fooled. The use of the word serenity here means freedom from mental and emotional pain—and that is a good thing. Serenity in this instance does *not* mean the state of mind/being in which we are unaffected by the world around us. But some mistakenly believe that the goal of therapy, indeed the goal of life, is to be protected and insulated from our own and others' tribulations. The finest part of what makes us human is to be touched by the world, moved by it, in all its turbulence. Should we not weep when others are suffering or rejoice when others are happy? Would we ever be inspired to attempt to change things if we only bliss-out and serenely accept others' suffering? Would great injustices like slavery ever have been stopped if those who felt them to be wrong decided to serenely accept them as inevitable rather than fight for change? Perhaps in some instances we have the right to choose the serenity option. Certainly, when it concerns our own suffering, we may want to accept it to a certain extent—and view it as a growth opportunity. But when it comes to the suffering of others, we must feel compassion, and, if possible, help.

Belief

Spirituality is an integral part of psychological well-being, but it isn't the sole focus of therapeutic treatment. We must recognize the coexistence of the spiritual (both positive and negative) and its partners—the mental and the emotional. We must also recognize the importance of the physical realms as we pursue wellness. However, actively exploring your spiritual self can fill in important gaps you may not even realize are there. Without belief in life's greater purpose, life loses much of its joy.

Many people believe their life's purpose is their career. Yet careers lack permanence. When some people lose their jobs, or they are no longer young enough to work, they are utterly devastated. We have all heard the stories about people who pass away shortly after retirement. Work was the only thing that gave their lives meaning. But it shouldn't be that way. Yes, work is meaningful, but many things give life meaning, including close relationships with family and friends, being part of a community, volunteering your time and giving to charity, developing your intellectual and artistic talents, appreciating the natural world, and so on. And, of course, your relationship with the God of your understanding also gives life meaning—many would argue its deepest meaning.

It has been our experience that those who believe in God (or a higher power of their own understanding) believe that their own lives are of great and lasting value. They tend to be able to make difficult changes while retaining hope, trust, and faith in the general goodness of the world. They intuit that there is a greater truth than what is visible to the senses—even though they may not be able to describe exactly what that truth is.

We want to clarify that we aren't talking about slavishly following a religion in a cultlike fashion or being controlled or brainwashed. What we are talking about is taking your spirituality seriously, basing life's choices on foundational moral codes that offer clarity, and finding a sense of belonging with others who feel the way you do.

The Pew Social Trends poll, which the Pew Research Center has been taking for more than thirty years, shows that adults who attend religious services at least once a week are consistently much more likely to report being happy than those who don't. The results show that 43 percent of these people are happy as compared to 26 percent of nonattendees! Again, we want to stress that we are not advocating you pursue a particular religious belief; we just want to stress the importance of exploring spirituality and having an understanding of what your foundational beliefs are.

Gabriel's Belief

Gabriel, unlike most of us, is very sick. He has schizophrenia, obsessive-compulsive disorder, and other complicating factors. Despite the help of powerful medications (which have severe side effects and are possibly shortening his life span), he suffers from violently upsetting auditory **hallucinations** *(imaginary voices or sounds that seem very real to the patient and can seem to come from inside his head, or outside in the general environment) and* **command hallucinations** *(a form of auditory hallucination where the imaginary voice or voices command the patient to generally do destructive or dangerous behaviors). He reacts to these and other internal stimuli whenever he is under stress—and any new or confusing event is stressful for him. To Gabriel, a stressful situation might mean he has to sit in a different chair than he usually does or might mean that he hears a bus driver and a rider argue when he's riding a public bus. He has had to be sedated and hospitalized many, many times, unfortunately.*

Yet Gabriel, who I have known for nine years, is a great role model and an inspiration. That's because he never gives up on goodness and never gives up on his conviction that the world is essentially a good place. When he was a boy, he was an excellent student of above-average intelligence, but today he can't concentrate for more than a brief time on any subject. Numerous times he has tried and failed to pass the GED (the high school degree equivalency exam). Each time he fails, he suffers great inner turmoil. "But," he will say to anyone who will listen, "I know it's for the best. I'll study harder, and with God's help, I'll pass next time."

Gabriel is also longing to get married. He comes from a large family and has many nephews and nieces. He feels that his siblings are getting on with life and that he is being left behind. He also feels time is running out—he is nearly forty. But he doesn't let this stop him. He fights against depression, perhaps harder than anyone I have ever met. He simply refuses to feel sorry for himself.

He attends social events for people with mental illness and introduces himself to women there. He shares, with whoever will listen, his hopes and dreams of marriage and raising a family. So far, he hasn't found someone to marry, but that doesn't stop him from trying to find his soul mate. He has faced more rejection than any of us can possibly imagine.

Gabriel is also longing to go to college. His dream is to be a psychologist. Yet he is unable, as mentioned, to pass the GED. But ask his roommates who they go to for help with problems, and they won't hesitate to tell you the answer: Gabriel. He brokers mini peace deals between his friends and offers his shoulder to cry on. He puts up with others' bad tempers and forgives very real offenses quite readily. He hasn't turned off his desire to help others because of his own suffering or because his own treasured goals seem to be unattainable. He reaches out and helps others whenever he can.

Gabriel's belief in the underlying good nature of people and this world fuels his ability to repeatedly transcend a debilitating illness that will most likely affect him the rest of his life. Despite moments of great suffering, Gabriel is often at peace because he believes that the challenges he has to face give his life meaning.

Some people who don't believe in a higher power seem to see the world as an essentially meaningless place where actions don't beget anything deeper than equally meaningless reactions. That kind of neutrality is a thinly disguised way of saying that the world is a bad empty place. By subscribing to *nihilism* (in psychotherapy, this refers to the delusion or misperception of reality that posits that the patient himself doesn't really exist), one is saying that nothing one does really matters. If nothing one does matters, why not just do whatever feels good, even if it hurts ourselves or others? If our desires dictate our choices and all options are equally meaningless, then the difference between good and evil isn't important—or even real.

However, our experience has been that the vast majority of people believe that what they do actually does matter. They have a sense of foundational morals and ethics, which is necessary for healthy self-esteem and healthy relationships with others. Morality and ethics certainly belong to the spiritual realm, but they can and must be an important discussion in therapy. It can be said that patients enter therapy to find a path to wellness and once in therapy learn they must actively fight against despair and darkness. When they follow through, they are choosing to participate in the creation of goodness and light.

Chapter 10

WHEN AND HOW TO MOVE ON

Character cannot be developed in ease and quiet. Only through experience of trial and suffering can the soul be strengthened, ambition inspired, and success achieved.

—HELEN KELLER

At some point you and your therapist will decide it is time for you to move on.

Patient: Doc, how will I know when therapy is over?

Therapist: When your insurance runs out.

Are you laughing? You shouldn't be! You and your therapist should plan a therapy budget and stick to it. Then your bank account and your mortgage will remain intact. It is possible that your therapist will initially recommend more therapy than you feel you can afford. We may have said this ad infinitum, but we want to be very clear—unless you have been diagnosed with a severe problem, you most likely will not need long-term, expensive therapy.

It's possible that your therapist may ask you to continue on in therapy after you have reached the end of the projected treatment time frame mentioned in your treatment plan. Ask your therapist the following: *Why do you recommend more therapy? What goals haven't I accomplished from my treatment plan? Please give me a clinical reason for the need for me to continue.* If you have found an ethical, competent, and caring therapist, he may very well have excellent reasons for having suggested more therapy. However, therapy will usually have ended when you have met the objectives and goals in your treatment plan.

I believe that together you and your therapist should figure out when it is really time to move on. That doesn't seem to be happening as much as it should. For example, in a 2008 study, 84 percent of the patients interviewed said they initiated the termination of therapy. Were they more in tune with when it was time to end therapy than their therapists?

Those patients in the study who said therapy ended too soon said that they felt forced to end it because it was too expensive for them or because they felt the therapist was a mismatch. Twenty-three percent of therapy patients in the study felt therapy lasted too long. Those patients reported that they stayed on because they hoped treatment would improve, or because they felt they themselves allowed it to go on too long, or because they felt dependent on the therapist and were afraid to leave. Of course, you must have a realistic view of whether or not you fulfilled your part of the bargain.

Erica: Resistance to Recommendations

Erica was nineteen years old when she came to see Francine, a colleague of mine, at her parents' request. She was having some severe problems. Francine gave her a thorough evaluation and recommended therapy twice a week for an initial period of six months, though she believed that Erica would require at least a year of therapy. Erica agreed—she was depressed, anxious, and worried about her own risky behavior. Her parents, on the other hand, refused and said they were only willing to send her to therapy twice a month. Although Francine recommended that they take Erica to a clinic where therapy would be less expensive or covered by their insurance so that she could get the recommended frequency of therapy, they balked—they were very concerned about anonymity. So Francine reluctantly took Erica on as a patient, hoping that as they worked together, Erica's parents would see the wisdom in the initial treatment frequency recommendations and comply.

Francine also recommended that the entire family see a marriage and family counselor to address family issues involving alcohol and physical abuse. The parents ignored her recommendations. Despite their professed commitment to having Erica go to therapy twice a month, Erica only showed up for six sessions over the course of seven months. Francine spent hours on the phone, unpaid, in conference with Erica's parents about the seriousness of her problems. But they refused to seriously address Erica's problems (or their own) and repeatedly refused to follow Francine's recommendations. Sadly, Francine terminated therapy knowing that continuing on in this way would not benefit Erica or her parents.

A competent therapist can generally motivate a patient to attend therapy, but it isn't always possible to motivate reluctant parents or guardians who are responsible for bringing a patient to treatment. Usually a competent therapist like Francine terminates therapy when a patient *has reached her goals.* In this case, Francine had no choice but to end therapy that was failing. Being a responsible therapist, Francine researched and suggested other therapists for Erica and her family to consider after she told them she would no longer be able to work with Erica.

Realistic Review

When we see that a course of therapy is drawing to a close, I like to sit with my patients and do a final, comprehensive review of their treatment plans. Of course, you and your therapist will have been reviewing your treatment plan all along, but when it appears that your major goals and objectives have been achieved, I believe a more detailed review is in order. As you strive to reach your goals, as well as after you reach them, it's important to ask some deeper questions, such as (1) *Has working on/completing these goals led me to develop insight into my thoughts, feelings, behaviors, and actions?* and (2) *Do I now have a solid ability to internalize and apply the concepts I have learned in therapy?*

Even if you have met your goals, if you haven't developed insight into your problems along the way, you are missing out on an important part of therapy. Of course, very simple goals may not necessitate such deep insights. Let's simplify: Therapy is like a car wash. Sure, you can get the superdeluxe, hand-applied, hot-wax, rustproof, tire-shine treatment, but the plain old wash-and-wipe will get you cleaned up and back on the road in half the time. Remember Grady? We could have spent time figuring out why he turned to caffeine when he was tired, or we could have explored whether or not he was allowing his employer to take advantage of him and dump too much work on his shoulders. But Grady wanted to simply address his anxiety—and together, we addressed it. Yes, we could have dug deeper and asked more questions about his reliance on stimulants, work pressures, and home life. However, there was no real, deep-seated need for longer-term therapy. We can all learn from Grady: *we don't have to achieve emotional perfection to live good and meaningful lives.*

At the risk of shocking those therapy gurus who would have you spend your lifetime (and your hard-earned dollars) in therapy, I believe, "If it ain't broke, don't fix it." Once you have achieved your goals, you can decide if you would like to pursue any ancillary issues or subgoals. Are you satisfied with where you are holding? Or would you like to dig deeper? Only you can decide if you want to spend more time and money on therapy.

When a patient and I decide it is time to move on, I think it's a great time to write or record a final PPP. You, too, may want to describe the internal and external changes that have occurred over the course of therapy. You may want to talk about not only your progress but also your doubts or fears, areas of concern, or ideas about where to go from here. By articulating your view of your therapy experience and your plans for the future, you will be able to assess how successful you feel the outcome has been. By describing your experience and sharing your insights and plans with your therapist, you give him additional information that can help him determine if his views of your progress and yours generally align. This will help him ensure that you have really progressed. Even though your therapist may not have used a PPP-type tool before, if the idea appeals to you, you might want to suggest it. Don't worry—your final PPP doesn't have to be time-consuming; it can be a page or two, and you can write or record it at home. Then discuss it briefly, during your final session, if you like.

Discharge Plan

Whether it has lasted weeks or months, your relationship with your carefully chosen, qualified therapist has most likely helped you in ways that differ dramatically from other professional and personal relationships in your life. Therapy should have helped you develop or refine your belief system, which will help you sustain the positive changes you have made. To make sure those positive changes will continue to be implemented in your life, your therapist and you should work on a *discharge plan*.

The discharge plan (in this instance, a plan created by a therapist and patient to help guide the patient after completing psychotherapy) actually begins to be written when your initial treatment plan is written. By planning for the end of therapy at the beginning, your therapist can get a deeper sense of where you want to be and what kind of support you will need to get there. The discharge plan will list the life areas you need to continue to work on after therapy, during *aftercare*. Remember, you are not a passive participant in aftercare, any more than you were during therapy. Aftercare will require your active participation in managing the people, places, and things in your life and includes the activities, therapies, and so on that are put in place to help you after you conclude psychotherapy—but you will still have to be an environmental warrior.

When training other therapists, I caution them that success in therapy is determined by the degree to which their patients will be able to internalize and apply what they've learned in therapy whenever they encounter rough spots in their lives. Remember: *wherever there is dysfunction, there is opportunity for growth*. And everybody has at least some dysfunction in their lives. Those initial areas of dysfunction you came into therapy with, and have hopefully resolved for the most part, will be listed in your discharge plan. So will any areas you still need to work on. Most important, the discharge plan will contain various recommendations that support the continued living out of your past, present, and future goals. Like your treatment plan, your discharge plan should be developed in collaboration with you. It will contain:

1. A patient self-report that discusses how confident you are that you can maintain therapeutic goals.
2. A relapse prevention plan. Usually this is a list of several actions that you can take to help you maintain your achievements, and will include specific activities that support wellness. Your relapse prevention plan may include or may be listed separately from numbers 3, 4, and 5 below.
3. An evaluation of the significant relationships in your life and how you can access them for support—the more you have the support of those close to you, the better you will do.
4. An evaluation of the need for professional support services such as group therapy, social agencies, ongoing medical/mental/emotional care, vocation-rehabilitation services, employment services, educational services, and environmental services.
5. Specific referrals to professionals and services.

You should receive a copy of your discharge plan when it is completed. Be sure to ask questions—it is essential for you to understand your discharge plan. The success of your aftercare will depend on your ability to comprehend and follow your discharge plan.

Discharge Summary and Treatment Records

There is another discharge document that will be written up, but you will most likely never see it. You should be aware that after you leave therapy, your therapist will write up a *discharge summary*. The discharge summary contains details of a patient's care, including initial diagnosis, course of treatment, progress, and outcome for the therapist's records, insurance information, or to help a therapist review a case in order to further help a former patient. It will include:

- Your initial and discharge diagnosis
- The reason for treatment
- A description of the clinical course of treatment
- The results of treatment
- The reason for discharge
- Recommendations and specific referrals

Another reason for the creation of a discharge summary is that your therapist may want a record for insurance purposes. The summary is a record of a completed (or sometimes incomplete) course of therapy. Additionally, like all therapists, yours should keep track of his therapeutic outcomes. The way he can do this is by following up with you and referring to your discharge summary when he does so. It will help him remember the details of your case and where you were holding when therapy was terminated.

I believe all therapists should know their successful outcome rates and base them not only on information gathered right after discharge but also for some time afterward. Your therapist will probably call you in a week or month or two to check in with you and see how you are doing. He may even ask you if he can contact you at the end of a year. By being candid with him about how you are feeling and how well you are fulfilling your plan for aftercare, you can help him become a better therapist. If a therapist finds that his outcomes are repeatedly poor, he should get more education, supervision, or reconsider the area of psychotherapy he is in. Perhaps he should consider another specialty.

It is also important that your therapist should call you at the very least once after your discharge because he genuinely cares about you and wants to see how you are doing. You may want to discuss some of your aftercare plans with him or get some advice. You may feel you need to come back in for a session or two. Or hopefully you will be able to tell him how great you are doing!

Remember all those notes your therapist took during (and after) your sessions? These notes are important records of your treatment and not only have clinical value, but also ethical/legal value. You may want a copy of these records for yourself. If you do, don't hesitate to ask. Also, if you go to another doctor or agency regarding a related problem, they may want to review your treatment records—but don't worry; it's illegal for your therapist to release your treatment records without your written permission.

Partners in Aftercare

One of the most important tasks that should take place during therapy is the development of your *personal support network,* which should include individual family members, friends, advisors, organizations, or other individuals or groups that can be supportive of a person during recovery and beyond. Sometimes a spouse or other family members (or close friends) may need to be taught to be understanding and supportive of you during and after therapy. They may have joined you for some psychoeducation. If that is so, they'll be able to see you through a new lens, and be able to recognize that they are dealing with a "new person"; not the difficult person who is hard to understand, but one with a set of struggles who is working to overcome them. Generally, family members of those with mental illness or addiction problems are themselves suffering. They find the stress of coping with a mentally ill or addicted family member to be overwhelming. They themselves might be struggling with substance abuse or emotional problems.

Studies show that the probability for continuing therapeutic success goes up dramatically with the development of a healthy, strong, and compassionate support network. After therapy, caring partners in your support network can give you tips and pointers about how to solve problems that come up. They can remind you to use techniques you learned during therapy. This can make an enormous impact on your continued wellness.

Therapeutic success does not happen in a vacuum. I know from keeping track of my own case outcomes: those patients with very supportive family members tend to do better over the long term than those patients without. Sometimes, though, in the real world, family members' own issues may impair their ability to help you. Even if your family is not so supportive, you can still do very well as long as you develop another kind of support network.

One of the benefits of joining a 12-step program or other support group is the chance to make friends who really understand what you are going through and can help you continue to achieve your goals. After therapy, there will be surprises, challenges, and new problems that will test your resolve and your ability to apply your newfound emotional skills to new situations.

Everybody needs a friend, companion, or mentor who can help them face life's challenges. Your therapist shouldn't become that type of support. The kind of intense support your therapist gives you *must* end in a reasonable time frame otherwise your therapist becomes part of the problem. In ancient China, the upper classes paid doctors to keep them well. If they became sick, the doctor wasn't paid until he cured them! The more a patient saw his doctor, the less the doctor was paid.

Though we operate somewhat differently today, we can borrow the general idea. Your therapist's job is to help you get to the point where you can function in an emotionally healthy way—without the need to see him. Sure, occasionally you may want to call your therapist to ask a question or two. But healthy, nontherapy relationships with family and friends with whom you can bare your soul and get—and give—feedback are essential to living a normal, healthy life.

There is an American cultural phenomenon where people's relationships with their therapists are taking the place of relationships with family and friends. I know it exists in big cities on both coasts; I am willing to bet that it exists to some extent in other places in the country. Remember, unless you have a serious problem, you should not be in therapy year after year. I strongly question the agenda of a therapist who would keep a patient in therapy for so long. Without knowing the particulars, it is hard to say definitively, but it would be a reasonable guess that some therapists view their patients as "paychecks."

If you haven't developed the ability to end therapy and live independently after a reasonable treatment time frame, ask yourself: *Why not? Why hasn't my therapist helped me develop the kind of skills I need to help me find and sustain interpersonal relationships?* Skill building of all kinds must be a part of good therapy. A therapist must help you make a life for yourself—a real life, without therapy. Also, the existence of a reasonable time frame for ending therapy, along with a comprehensive discharge plan that clearly outlines your support network, shows that your therapist wants you to succeed without him.

On Your Own:
Self-Caring Versus Selfishness

For therapeutic purposes, we define these two terms in the following way: *self-caring* is the process by which a person develops awareness of and strives to satisfy real physical, emotional, intellectual, and spiritual needs while taking into consideration the needs of others. *Selfishness* is the state in which a person strives to satisfy perceived needs and desires without taking into account the needs of others.

There can be many variations of self-caring and selfishness, and sometimes it may be important for you to be a little bit of both. For example, a person can be aware of his own very real needs but allow the desires of others to take precedence—this may or may not be healthy, depending on the situation. Or a person can work to satisfy his own real needs but utterly ignore the needs of others—again, this may or may not be healthy. Although many philosophical ramifications of these two approaches can be explored, suffice it to say that a person in recovery from mental/emotional problems and/or substance abuse/addiction must learn to care for himself. He must be able to strike a balance between his own need to stay well and the demands of relationships and of life in general. He must learn to negotiate these differences and reach a practical compromise without compromising his wellness. It can be a tightrope walk.

Someone who is so distracted by others, perhaps because he cares so much about others that he is willing to do things that would be harmful to his recovery, must compel himself to act somewhat selfishly. In this instance, he may have to ignore the needs of others when making decisions. Indeed, it is common for someone who is in the early stages of struggling with a mental illness or addiction to act in this manner, at least for a while.

With those who would compromise his wellness, he must either stand firm and set healthy boundaries or limit contact. The most obvious example would be someone who is a recovering alcoholic. If his friends want him to join them in a bar, and he knows that the atmosphere would trigger his cravings, he mustn't go. If these friends keep on pressing him to join them, he will have to find new friends. He must be somewhat selfish in order to be self-caring.

Mark, who we learned about earlier in Chapter 5, no longer lives at home with his parents. In order to manage his depression, he has committed himself to exercising five days a week for an hour each time. The exercise has helped him reduce medications. His schedule, however, only allows him to exercise after work each day at 5:00 in his company's gym. His coworkers are annoyed that Mark won't carpool with them, but he is standing firm. He knows that he must exercise, though he is happy to give a ride to whoever needs one, if they will hang around until 6:00.

This basic chart (Figure 10.1) may help you understand various components of self-caring and selfishness. Remember: sometimes you may have to be selfish!

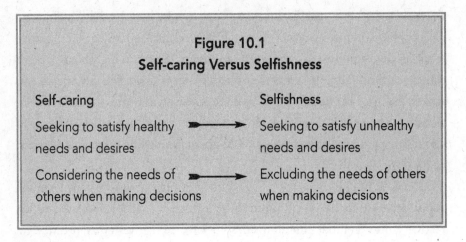

Figure 10.1
Self-caring Versus Selfishness

Self-caring		Selfishness
Seeking to satisfy healthy needs and desires	➤	Seeking to satisfy unhealthy needs and desires
Considering the needs of others when making decisions	➤	Excluding the needs of others when making decisions

Let's take another example. You and your therapist may decide that after therapy has been terminated, you need to include journal writing as part of your self-care program. You decide it is important for you to write in your journal each evening. One evening your sister says, "Hey, let's go to the mall." You know that if you don't get to your journal right away, you probably won't go back to it later. You'll be skipping an entire day of journal writing. Is it so terrible? It's not like you are doing something overtly detrimental to your health. Your sister is pressuring you: "Stop being so selfish." When you hear the buzzword "selfish" (you may hear it often—at least for a while after you are discharged from therapy), that may mean it is time to slow down and pay attention. Are you really being selfish, trying to satisfy desires, not constructive needs? Or are you trying to meet a very real need, one that will keep you on the path to wellness? You will now have to make these important decisions on your own. You will have to assume personal responsibility for your choices.

Responsibility, Suffering, and Time

Accepting personal responsibility for your choices can sometimes be somewhat daunting—for anyone. However, it is also liberating. It frees you from the blame game. It frees you from feeling powerless. It frees you from immaturity. It is virtually a given that in psychotherapy you will touch on the subject of taking responsibility for your feelings, actions, and behaviors in some measure. And you will learn the parameters of personal responsibility as well, such as that described in the "Serenity Prayer." Blending humility with action is a hard lesson, but one well worth learning.

But taking personal responsibility for things can be overwhelming. So how do you take responsibility without totally collapsing under the weight of it all? By limiting your attempts to one day, one hour, or even one minute at a time. Sometimes people can't live on a daily basis, so they have to live on an hourly basis, or a minute-by-minute basis. You may be suffering from anxiety. Depression. An addiction. You may have reached your basic treatment goals but now you want or need to move on. Perhaps you are just scaling back your therapy from weekly sessions to monthly sessions. No matter what point you are at in therapy or after therapy, you might need to bite off small chunks of time and chew them well, versus biting off bigger chunks and choking on the pieces.

In order to act responsibly, avoiding things that can derail your mental/emotional wellness, you might have to view time like this. It may be easier to not give in to a craving, or sadness, or anxiety if you fight it just for this minute and the next. Hopefully, your symptoms will have abated so much that this isn't an issue for you. But if it is an issue for you, remember: take charge of your minutes and build on them.

A word of caution: Just because you are dealing with time and personal responsibility in this way—and perhaps combating bad feelings—doesn't mean that you automatically still need to be in therapy. You may have to struggle like this for a while with the help of your support network and other measures from your discharge plan. That's okay. Your therapist should have taught you as many ways as you need to manage your symptoms.

There are therapists out there who would keep patients in therapy five days a week, year after year if they could. They provide patients with so much structure, so many restrictions, that they can't begin to see their way toward independence. I am not talking about patients with serious mental illnesses (and even they need to develop more independence than this); I am talking about people like you who end up addicted to therapy, on therapy welfare, stuck in the endless therapy trap. If you are reading this chapter because you think you are at the point where therapy should have ended but hasn't, speak directly to your therapist. Be frank. Say something like, "I am really convinced that I am able to and need to end therapy." Remember, if he says you still need to be in therapy, ask him specifically: "What are the clinical reasons why you believe I still need to be in therapy?" Be sure to write down his answers so you can remember them, research them, and discuss them with mentors and other wise friends. Your therapist may very well have reasonable and important clinical reasons at this point in time. However, it is important to keep in mind that the most basic goal of therapy is to help you live a mentally and emotionally healthy life without therapy.

Head to Heart

Early in recovery from any mental illness or addiction, a person simply can't trust his own feelings. You have to keep checking in with your therapist and members of your support network. *Is what I am feeling valid? How can I reconcile my feelings with what my intellect says is right?* Mental illness, addiction, and even most emotional problems are "feeling" diseases. They are diseases of self-deception. *By allowing your diseased feelings to determine your choices, you will end up sucked into a spiral of negativity.*

Let your anatomy be your guide here. Your head (intellect) is above your heart (feelings). Therefore, your very body has been designed with a message: Let your head lead—after all, it's on top, above the heart. You have to use your intellect to harness your feelings and steer them toward the right path. It doesn't mean you should suppress your feelings. It doesn't mean you should ignore your feelings. It does mean that your feelings can't blossom fully until they are refined and used for a higher purpose.

With very overwhelming feelings, especially cravings, rage, or despair, you may want to imagine that your feelings are like an ocean. If you can't manage your feelings at this point, you can "ride them out." Visualize the feelings as waves and you as the surfer. Don't get sucked into the swirling water; ride your feelings out until they reach the shore, lapping gently at the sand. Of course, your therapist should have taught you as many techniques as you need to master in order to face the challenges life brings.

Commencement

When you graduate from high school and college, you receive your diploma during a ceremony called "commencement." Although your therapist isn't going to hand you a diploma, in a very real sense, graduating from therapy is a "commencement"—a new beginning. Though recovery is a process, not a onetime event, leaving therapy and gaining independence is a momentous occasion. But as we said in the beginning of this book, just because you are done with therapy doesn't mean you will never have to suffer again. You will experience pain—we all do. But the suffering you experience now will be qualitatively (and hopefully quantitatively) different than the sensations you experienced before treatment, because now you are armed with the skills to resolve self-defeating behaviors, you've learned ways to manage internal and external challenges, and you are able to view painful experiences as growth opportunities. Your problems now, after therapy, will be problems of living with awareness. These problems are part of healing, too.

How many times has Gabriel, our dear friend with schizophrenia, not been able to hold his ground? Too many to count. His illness isn't one that can be cured—at least, not yet. His periods of suffering wax and wane. Most of the rest of us have a less intense experience of life's challenges. And that's the way we want it. Now, like Gabriel, we are hopefully able to live with our problems and see them, at least sometimes, as gifts.

Healing Yourself

This book has been about how to hire a great therapist. It has given you tips and pointers and lists. It has given you a general overview of what you can expect from an ideal therapy experience. It has suggested specific activities such as interviews, research, and ideas about what questions to ask your therapist about the therapy process itself. Essentially, this book has been about how to advocate for yourself as well as take responsibility for your own therapy experience. By researching, interviewing, assessing, evaluating, discussing, questioning, and suggesting, you have taken charge of your therapy experience. By being a savvy consumer of therapy, you have learned how to actively be involved in healing yourself. Now thats good therapy.

Bibliography

Books

American Psychiatric Association. *Diagnostic and Statistical Manual of Mental Disorders-IV-TR (DSM-IV-TR)*. 4th ed. Arlington, VA: American Psychiatric, 2000.

Anonymous. *The AA Big Book*. 4th ed. New York: Alcoholics Anonymous World Services, 2002.

Corey, Gerald. *Theory and Practice of Counseling and Psychotherapy*. 8th ed. Pacific Grove, CA: Brooks Cole, 2008.

Egan, Gerard. *The Skilled Helper: A Problem-Management and Opportunity-Development Approach to Helping*. 9th ed. Pacific Grove, CA: Brooks Cole, 2009. *[In our opinion, and in the opinion of many experienced therapists, Gerard Egan's "The Skilled Helper" texts are the ones that started the most important therapy revolution more than two decades ago. Dr. Egan, retired professor of psychology and organizational studies at Loyala University in Chicago, wisely posits that the only therapy worth doing is therapy that actually produces results.]*

Eysenck, Michael W. *Simple Psychology*. New York: Taylor & Francis, 1996.

Twerski, Abraham J., M.D. *Generation to Generation: Personal Recollections of a Chassidic Legacy*. United Kingdom: CIS International, 1986.

Wegscheider-Cruse, Sharon. *Another Chance: Hope and Health for the Alcoholic Family*. Palo Alto, CA: Science and Behavior Books, 1981.

Wineberg, Yosef. *Lessons in Tanya (The Tanya of R. Schneur Zalman of Liadi)*. 3rd printing. New York: Kehot Publication Society, 1996.

Articles, Studies, and Statistics

Miller, William R., Ph.D., and William White, M.A. "Confrontation in Addiction Treatment." *Counselor Magazine*, October, 2007. http://www.counselor-magazine.com/content/view/608/63.

Office of the Professions. New York State Department of Education, 2006.

Roe, David, Rachel Dekel, Galit Harel, and Shmuel Fennig. "Sixty Percent of Psychotherapy Clients Felt Therapy Didn't End on Time." *ScienceDaily*, University of Haifa, January 10, 2008. http://www.sciencedaily.com/releases/2008/01/080109094351.htm.

U.S. Department of Health and Human Services. National Survey on Drug Use and Health National Findings. Substance Abuse and Mental Health Services Administration (SAMHSA), Office of Applied Studies, 2006.

Websites

www.afriprov.org (African proverbs)

www.amhca.org

www.apa.org

www.bartleby.com (quotations)

www.bls.gov

www.op.nysed.gov

www.psych.org

www.samhsa.org

Resources

Authors' website: Therapyrevolutiononline.com

Individual State Government Mental Health and Addiction Agencies
The most important resource about psychotherapists in your area is your own state government mental health and addiction agencies. At state government websites you may find links to your state agencies/offices of mental health, alcoholism, and drug abuse. Ask them what licenses and certifications are required in your state and ask them where you can find current lists of practitioners whose licenses are up-to-date.

Substance Abuse and Mental Health Services Administration (SAMHSA)
This national agency belongs to the United States Department of Health and Human Services. It is an excellent, no-nonsense source of comprehensive information about mental health and addiction. www.samhsa.gov.

12-Step Programs
These sites offer free self-help meetings in your area; check online. Remember, these programs offer excellent recovery and support networks, but they are not a cure or treatment for addictions:
Alcoholics Anonymous: www.aa.org
Gamblers Anonymous: gamblersanonymous.org
Narcotics Anonymous: www.na.org
Overeaters Anonymous: www.oa.org

Programs for families of those with addictions
Al-Anon, Alateen, Nar-Anon, Gam-anon, and so on.

Professional Associations:
Professional associations can be a good source of information about specific types
of psychotherapy. We have included just a few of the major groups—there are several others. Most association/group websites have search functions that can help
you find a practitioner in your area. Remember, the lists that professional associa-
tions give you are almost always not personalized referrals or recommendations;
they are lists of professionals who meet the requirements of memberships and
belong to their organization.
American Association for Marriage and Family Therapy: www.aamft.org
American Mental Health Counselors Association: www.amhca.org
American Psychiatric Association: www.psych.org
American Psychological Association: www.apa.org
American Society of Group Psychotherapy & Psychodrama: www. asgpp.org
National Association of Social Workers: www.naswdc.org

Patients' Advocacy Organization:
National Alliance on Mental Illness
The website www.nami.org is a good source of information for people with mental
illness and their families.

Index

About the Authors

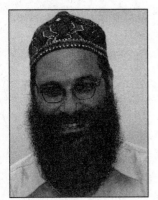

Richard M. Zwolinski, LMHC, CASAC, SAP, ADS, ICADC, is a nationally and internationally licensed psychotherapist and addiction specialist. He is a consultant to government and nongovernmental agencies and industries, and is a regulatory compliance officer and director of a clinical treatment program. He also has a private psychotherapy practice and speaks to organizations and businesses about mental health and addiction.

Richard serves on the New York State OASAS Administrative Regulatory Relief Committee and is involved in the creation of important patients' rights regulations. He is also the provider co-chair for the OASAS Smart Records Committee and helping to develop systems designed to keep patients engaged in treatment while promoting therapists' adherence to treatment protocols. He also serves on the Ethics Committee for the New York State Mental Health Counselors Association.

Whenever he is able, he enjoys basketball, swimming, running, and martial arts as well as volunteering with youth-at-risk. He lives in Brooklyn, NY.

C.R. Zwolinski is a writer and editor. She volunteers her time teaching whole-foods cooking to those with chronic illnesses.

Please visit the Therapy Revolution website to view the authors' blog and to learn more about the therapy process: www.therapyrevolution online.com.